The Energy Advantage

Fuelling Your Body and Mind for Success

Dr Christine Fenn

Thorsons
An Imprint of HarperCollins*Publishers*

Thorsons
An Imprint of HarperCollins*Publishers*
77–85 Fulham Palace Road,
Hammersmith, London W6 8JB
1160 Battery Street
San Francisco, California 94111–1213

Published by Thorsons 1997
10 9 8 7 6 5 4 3 2

A catalogue record for this book
is available from the British Library

ISBN 0 7225 3377 2

Printed and bound in Great Britain by
Caledonian International Book Manufacturing Ltd Glasgow

To
Mum, Dad, Richard and Caroline.
The Angels who will take you on a special journey
and teach you how to fly – if you let them.

Contents

Acknowledgements

First to Jean for her friendship and patience in reading every page of the raw manuscript, tossing out the extra words and rearranging whole sentences to make my ideas flow freely. My thanks to Carole, my editor at Thorsons, for her encouragement, support and expertise.

Introduction

Ask yourself how you feel right now? If the answer is 'pretty whacked' or 'could be better' the chances are your energy levels are low.

Number one on the *Harvard Business Review's* list of essential qualities for business success is 'a high level of drive and energy'. In *The Energy Advantage* I show you how you can gain large and incredible health benefits by making just small changes to your diet and lifestyle – and at the same time give a significant boost to your energy levels so that you have the edge on your rivals.

The energy factor is a common denominator in all successful people, and to hear them talk with such drive and passion, you would think that at least they were born with an extra pint of blood, or had pure adrenalin continually pumping through their veins. Their secret is simply that they have the power to think positively and the stamina to pursue their goals.

The key to it all, then, is to be found in the mind – but you will miss the point if you see the mind in isolation. What originates in your brain – your thoughts, feelings and fears – has an immediate knock-on effect on the rest of you. What better example of this than when you are called upon to stand up and give a presentation. You try to remain calm but your heart pounds, your hands go sweaty and your mouth feels so dry that you can hardly speak!

Such signals are two way – your body can also influence your mind. Premenstrual syndrome can send emotions and irritability levels sky high; when you hug someone you care about, a soothing rush of warmth makes you feel good. These effects result from a release of messenger molecules called neuropeptides. When triggered by emotions, they send a variety of signals which alter the metabolism of your entire body.

The characteristic positive attitude and passion for life of successful people keeps these beneficial neuropeptides flowing. This generates a flood of internal energy which makes them believe that they can achieve anything – and they do!

Anita Roddick, founder of the Body Shop, has an energy level that is legendary. Her success is based on her passionate belief that her idea, to sell a range of beauty products made from natural ingredients, would work. It did! The Body Shop is now a £280 million concern, sporting 1,300 branches in 45 countries. Similarly, Tracey Edwards needed energy and stamina to keep her mind fixed firmly on the path to her goal – to skipper the first all-female crew in the Whitbread Round The World Yacht Race. She tirelessly kept knocking on the doors of potential sponsors, not only to find money but also to find a boat!

Not everyone can be, or even wants to be, the first at anything or a record-breaking entrepreneur, but having a positive outlook generates energy – which means reaching your full potential, finding your own success and being all you can be. It's a competitive world – in business at all levels we need to have the edge so that we remain one step ahead of our rivals. This is why we need to develop a passion, have goals and the drive to push ourselves that little bit further and enjoy the success that this brings. With the energy advantage those vital contracts are signed, sales are closed, deals are done and promotion achieved.

Endurance and optimism are also vital assets when things are not going so well. If you find you are pipped at the post by competitors, or made redundant, remember that it is the person with energy and self-belief who bounces back, again and again, with the conviction that next time will be better. Life is a challenge, and progress and achievement comes from falling down six times but being able to get up seven times. You must keep trying – using new approaches or new techniques. Competition in the business world is so intense that everyone, from the summit of management to the teams on the shop floor, needs to be fired by self-belief and constantly ready to change and adapt.

The most powerful force in the sporting world is not a professional team; it is a shoe company. Phil Knight, Managing Director of Nike, a reclusive, unpredictable entrepreneur turned a two-man operation, importing running shoes, into a $4 billion company. Employees routinely take two hours at lunchtime to exercise, enjoy a light meal, and then continue with schemes and creatively strategize late into the night to keep their competitive edge. Outsiders think Nike is a cult, but insiders are charged with a passion and a belief that they work for a company of the moment and one of the future. They are! By early 1993 one out of every three pairs of sports shoes sold in the US were Nikes.

Whatever your goals in life: to work more efficiently; think more creatively; achieve your full potential and pack more into each day without feeling constantly tired, you need the fundamental fuel. But, it seems that extreme tiredness, fatigue, exhaustion and lethargy are endemic today. As I travel around the world giving lectures and seminars, what amazes me is how often people ask the question 'How can I put the zip, zest and vitality back into my life?'

The paradox is that, as we drive ourselves harder each day, we neglect the importance of fuelling our bodies and feeding our minds. We grab poor quality fast foods and eat on the run – which only adds to the stress, and drains our energy reserves even further. The end result is that we are overfed and undernourished.

This is why this book has been written. Having worked in Nepal as the Expedition Nutritionist with the successful 1993 Everest expedition – which put Rebecca Stephens, MBE (first British woman to climb Everest), on the summit – I witnessed at first hand the power that food quality and good nutrition have on the mental and physical challenge of climbing to the highest point on earth. Many of the principles that I used in designing the diets for the climbers apply to the stress and challenge of achieving what we want in business, and I have included them in this book.

It will give you the inspiration, information and motivation to make the changes to your eating habits that will bring maximum energy into your life. The first part examines what it is about living in the nineties that leaves us so drained; our get up and go has certainly got up and gone! Part of the reason is that we have a warped idea of what a successful person should be like. It is someone who drives themselves unremittingly at a problem, striving to keep going for hours on end, then jumps onto a plane, hits the ground running and after a quick shower continues work on the other side of the world.

The quickest way to wear out a machine is to use it continually without pause for maintenance. The secret of successful living is to tune into the body's natural cycles of peak performance and repair. Chapter 3 explains the benefits of power napping and the profits to be gained from quality recovery time. You have to ask yourself which would you rather be, a live wire or a burnt out fuse?

There are plenty of ways to make changes. Think of all the negative aspects of your eating habits that drain your energy – drinking coffee, eating sugary snacks, gorging on saturated fats. It is time to toss these out and replace them with habits that will have a positive effect on your stamina and put the fizz back into each day.

Making these changes is the stumbling block for many of us. People find change uncomfortable and believe that benefits only come with denial, suffering and pain. How wrong! The exciting and the good news is that even the tiniest changes can make a dramatic difference. This book is specifically for busy people and is peppered with energizing principles broken up into bite-sized chunks. This means that you can put one or two simple ideas into practice at a time.

And they are so simple! Let's face it, they need to be if we are to fit them into our already busy and stressful lives. Although a degree of stress may give us a 'buzz', too much of it and we feel out of control. It is this lack of control which can drain our mental and physical energy. Too much stress results in you feeling harassed, nervous, time-pressured, angry and worn out. Phew! You need to take control of your lifestyle, gather your personal resources and begin to make the small changes that will put back the spark and vitality into each day and give you the energy advantage over those stuck in the energy drain.

A new-found optimism comes with renewed energy levels. You will find yourself looking on the bright side, mixing with people who see the glass half full, rather than those who moan that it is half empty. With the energy advantage your self-esteem will grow as you embrace change with enthusiasm and relish new challenges.

1

Eating for Energy – Stress and Fibre

Personal energy is something that many of us find to be in short supply, and we can only gasp in awe and envy at those who have it aplenty. Richard Branson is enviable, not only in his vision, sense of adventure and daring as a true entrepreneur, but also in his seemingly boundless energy with which he achieves success after success. Unfortunately for most people, each day will probably prove to be a survival exercise rather than a fulfilling experience.

It is natural to feel tiredness, but sheer exhaustion – being totally 'wrecked' and suffering from debilitating fatigue – seems to be more the norm in today's hectic world. The underlying cause is stress. We measure progress by the speed at which we get things done. City-dwellers have learned to walk, talk and eat faster; we are now 25 times more productive than we were 150 years ago – but it is not clear what we personally have actually gained. As the pace of living continues to increase, we continue to do more and strive to achieve more, seemingly forgetting that we are human beings, not human doings. As the pace of change intensifies, we may be in danger of trapping ourselves in an accelerating spiral of speed and stress. The thing about the rat race is that, even if you win it, you are still a rat at the end!

Fast Living and Fatigue

Because of the demands of work and family life, most of us rush through each day trying to keep too many balls in the air? Women dash out to work, but also have to find time to prepare meals, to shop, to ferry the children about and generally look after the family. Men are also under increasing pressure to put more and more time into their jobs.

We are working longer and trying to pack more into each day than ever before. Stress is coming at us from all angles. Reorganization within companies and the threat of redundancy creates a pressure-cooker environment in the workplace, and the workload heaped onto us each day is made the greater by the ever-increasing speed of communications. Not long ago you posted a letter and waited for a reply. Now there are faxes, mobile phones, pagers and e-mail.

So, we have a new breed of businessman and businesswoman – the workaholic. Are you one? Do you get up at five and work until midnight? Do you work more than you have to, take work home – or with you even when you are on 'holiday'? Workaholism has been called the respectable addiction. Its victims may be hardworking, motivated and ambitious by choice, but some are also driven, unhappy and caught in the trap of our modern, industrial society – where a smaller workforce is expected to cope with a larger workload.

A recent survey in Britain revealed that one in eight managers works more than 60 hours per week, and 40 per cent work more than 50 hours. Many more have forgotten the meaning of the word 'weekend' – doctors are on call, university lecturers use it to keep abreast of research, schoolteachers mark homework and prepare classes, salespeople plan their targets and the self-employed catch up with administration, stock control and book-keeping. We are heading full tilt into the 24-hour, 365-days a year, work routine and it is all made possible by information technology and the computer – there are no sunsets on the Internet.

Whatever the reasons, the price for living the life of a workaholic is high – a heart attack, a personal crisis or total burn-out in early or mid-life. Now is the time to ask yourself if it is all worth it? After all, nobody ever said on their deathbed: 'I wish I'd spent more time at the office.'

With such emphasis on work, eating well slips way down the priority list – if it appears at all. The often quoted axiom that breakfast is the most important meal of the day seems to fall on deaf ears, for just under half of us choose not to eat it – or at most have a drink of tea or coffee. We may have food in the kitchen but simply do not feel like eating anything. Does this matter? It does if you ate your last meal at 7 p.m., missed breakfast and had lunch at 1 p.m. – that's 18 hours without sustenance. There is no doubt that long periods between meals deplete the body of its glycogen energy reserves and, as a result, physical performance suffers.

The question for business people who are confined to a desk is whether mental performance is more effective if they eat breakfast? One study revealed that those who missed breakfast suffered from poorer memory and concentration later in the morning compared with those who did not. The effects of no breakfast were more pronounced when increased demands were put on the worker. It seems that if you are faced with a three-hour exam, extended meeting, or your job demands that you need to pay attention and act on a lot of continuous information, then eating breakfast would definitely prove helpful. This restores blood sugar levels to normal after the overnight fast and keeps your brain supplied with glucose.

Breakfast, however, means taking more than just an extra spoonful of sugar in your cup of coffee. The effect of a combination of caffeine and sugar first thing in the morning, when blood glucose levels are low, is to stimulate the production of insulin and adrenalin. Together these hormones work to stabilize the sudden rush of blood sugar from the drink, but ultimately the result is a roller coaster effect. Initially your blood sugar rises and you feel invigorated, but those sugar levels will soon come crashing down, starving your brain of vital fuel and prompting symptoms of hypoglycaemia – headache, despair, rapid pulse, irritability, mental confusion and forgetfulness. All this is not going to help you do your job, especially if you are a manager or business executive who has to be one step ahead of his or her competitors!

The best business breakfast combination is tea (herb, weak black or green tea), with either some carbohydrate food (bowl of porridge, toast with jam, honey, etc., piece of fruit) or protein food (pot of natural yogurt with chopped flaked almonds, scrambled, poached or boiled egg with tomato and mushrooms). More information about what to eat for maximum mental performance is given in later chapters.

Beat Stress – Build Success

In Britain, 40 million working days are lost each year through stress-related illness. British Airways estimates that stress accounts for 30 per cent of sick days; the Post Office reckons even higher at 40 per cent. Not surprisingly, many companies are keen to find ways to reduce stress and the effect it has on their workforces. For the individual, it is not the stress itself which is harmful, but how we perceive it. Stuck in a traffic jam, most of us feel stressed. It is not the traffic jam, but the voice inside your head telling you that you'll be late that does the damage. Make the voice tell you something different (that this is a time free of meetings and a chance to think), and you have triggered the chemical messages that have a positive effect on the body.

An optimistic outlook is just about the best energy booster and immunization against disease there is. The brain and the immune system constantly feed each other non-stop messages. Chemicals known as lymphokines are activated by the brain to help the body fight illness. Emotions such as happiness, hope, purpose, determination, faith and love prompt the brain to send positive immune-system-strengthening messages. Negative emotions, such as fear, anxiety, anger or depression, have the opposite effect.

The coexistence of stress and illness is no coincidence. There are plenty of signals that warn us that we are not coping well with stress – persistent headaches, colds and flu, backache, poor sleeping habits, teeth grinding, fainting or dizziness, a feeling of weakness and lacking in energy! They drive us to consult a doctor who may prescribe pills and antibiotics, but this does not deal with the underlying festering dis-ease. Duly medicated, we toss ourselves back into the fray until Mother Nature knocks again – with an ulcer or chest pains.

All in all, we do not cope well with stress. This is partly because the human system isn't geared towards twentieth century living. We have a stone age metabolism trying to cope with today's alien lifestyle. According to the social anthropologists, the species homo sapiens has spent the majority of its time on earth as hunter gatherers, living in mutually protective sociable groups. Nowadays work is an isolated activity spent mostly interacting with various bits of technology rather than real individuals. We no longer have to hunt for our food – instead we stalk the aisles of the supermarket for instant nourishment in the form of 'TV dinners' and microwave meals. No wonder we feel lonely and cut off – work and eating have become solitary activities. Without the social interaction that human beings crave, it is not surprising that we turn inwards and look to food and eating for comfort.

Unfortunately, no amount of comfort-eating can satisfy the need for companionship, sharing, nurturing and being nurtured in the same way that working with others, cooking and providing food in a group does. Instead, the most popular comfort foods (chocolate, chips, crisps, biscuits and ice-cream) have empty Calories and do little to nourish the body. The feelings of guilt and depression that tend to follow periods of comfort-eating, are amongst those negative emotions listed earlier that drain our energy and crush our immune system.

Fast Food – Sluggish System

In the demanding world of business and so-called progress, our eating habits (so often based on fast foods) have been distorted and mangled to fit around our hectic lifestyle – rather than being given a priority within it. With the next appointment to get to, there is no time to linger over an enjoyable meal. To keep up with the clock we must rely on fast foods and re-fuel on the run – or not at all!

Food manufacturers have created products to suit this lifestyle. Marks and Spencer alone produce a million pre-packed sandwiches each week, and the most popular filling is prawn cocktail. Is this entirely because of the taste and nutritional value? More likely it is because the ingredients stay firmly within the bread – essential if you have a sandwich in one hand and a phone or a steering wheel in the other. Hot dogs are another popular choice – again, not so much for the flavour but for the fact that the over-processed, plastic white bread can be moulded and squeezed securely onto the sausage inside. This is reassuring, as you know that it will not fall apart and make a mess whilst you are eating it. It allows you to switch off completely from the process of eating and mindlessly push food into your mouth whilst concentrating on other things.

It should be obvious, if we want to change our eating habits, that we need to change not only what we are consuming but how and why we eat it. Stress is the buzz word of the decade, and the popular saying, 'It's not what you eat, but what's eating you!', has never been more true than when accounting for the maladies of modern man and woman.

So, the first step that workaholics or business executives must take to gain the energy advantage is to take stock of their lives and regain a feeling of personal control. Experts agree that it is the loss of control which results in negative stress, and is responsible for draining our energy. This is when we reach for a cup of coffee to kick-start the system, or drown our emotions in alcohol. These actions are merely a sop for the brain, and in the long term can do more harm than good.

There are plenty of ways to regain that feeling of personal power. Taking action and making even the smallest changes to your eating and exercise habits will boost your self-esteem, confidence and energy levels. The current boom in alternative therapies (meditation, hypnotherapy, aromatherapy massage, yoga, flotation tanks) is an indication that many people are seeking an antidote to stress. The common denominator for all of these therapies is relaxation. Being more relaxed and in control will enable you to focus not only on WHAT to eat to give you more vitality, but on HOW to eat.

Good digestion is the root of health and vitality, and the gut is a barometer of the health of the rest of your body. Intestinal diseases signal that food is not being digested, and that the full range of nutrients in the food are not being absorbed into your body. Treat your intestines well by taking the time to chew food and by choosing foods that you have to chew! Such meals are sometimes difficult to find, but with careful choice it is possible to construct an energizing snack. Many fast food restaurants now offer salads, fruit, scones and baked potatoes as a healthy option to the high-fat burgers and pies. Whilst the occasional fast food meal is not out of the question, you will notice a big difference in your energy levels if you routinely aim to base meals and snacks on 'real' foods.

Fibre to the Rescue

'Real' foods are the high-fibre foods – as close as possible to their natural state. For example, sandwiches are wonderful mini-meals to graze on during the day; they fit in with our take-away, mobile style of living. But choose those made from a large wholemeal roll, filled with plenty of salad ingredients – lettuce, watercress, cucumber, bean sprouts, coleslaw, radish, celery, green and red pepper. Such a sandwich, to avoid the filling falling on your lap, needs both hands and demands your complete attention. It cannot be gulped down in less than a minute. It should be enjoyed and savoured to the full. Such food will provide your body with a range of nutrients, which will be fully absorbed, and with essential fibre, which is not absorbed.

Your grandmother may have called it 'roughage', but the new name for dietary fibre is non-starch polysaccharide (NSP). It cannot be broken down by our enzymes and so passes the entire length of our intestines (all 26 feet from mouth to anus), acting as a therapeutic bottle brush. Originally, because fibre was not absorbed (the contents of the intestines are considered to be 'outside' the body), it was considered worthless, and fibre was specifically removed from foods during processing and fed to animals! The modern Western diet then became fibre-free – and along with it came a host of intestinal disorders.

We now know a lot more about the function of fibre in the gut and its role in the prevention of diseases such as appendicitis, constipation, colon cancer and even heart disease. The power of fibre lies in the very fact that it is not digested by our enzymes but can absorb up to 15 times its weight of water. It is this bulk which is easily transported right through the intestine, taking any toxins that may have accumulated along with it.

Fibre – The Inside Story

Fibre is a type of carbohydrate which exists only in foods of plant origin, so you won't find it in eggs, meat, butter, oils, fish or dairy products. There are two main types of fibre – soluble and insoluble.

Soluble fibre is in apples, pears, bananas, peas, lentils, barley, porridge oats and all sorts of beans – kidney, baked beans, soya beans. It dissolves in water and becomes a gummy substance, rather like wallpaper paste. It is important in the stomach and upper intestine as it gives a feeling of fullness and helps to control the absorption of nutrients into the bloodstream. This results in a steady trickle of glucose into the body, keeping our energy levels topped up and those sugar cravings at bay. Highly processed fatty and sugary foods are concentrated sources of Calories. They are easy to eat (think of the time that it takes to eat a small bar of chocolate compared with a couple of apples), and easy to over-eat. If our diet is based on these highly processed foods, we soon put on weight. Isn't it crazy the way many of us then try to fight the flab? We think that eating less – practically starving ourselves – will make the pounds disappear, when eating a lot more low-fat, high-fibre foods will do the job more easily and enjoyably. The French and Mediterranean people know how to eat well and spend hours over a single meal! Their diet is bursting with high-fibre ingredients which people love to eat – whole roasted peppers and tomatoes stuffed with rice and marinaded in garlic, herbs and olive oil. Huge substantial salads with chunks of oven-baked crusty bread all served with freshly grilled fish steaks.

Insoluble fibre is more stringy and fibrous. It is found in celery and green leafy vegetables, but by far the richest source is wheat bran and wholegrain cereals. White flour has had the bran removed – so white bread provides much less fibre. If you had to make one change to increase the amount of fibre in your diet, the most effective would be to change from eating white bread, to wholemeal bread. This would significantly – but gently – increase your fibre intake. If you already enjoy wholemeal bread, aim to gradually increase your intake to six slices per day. If you find it difficult to eat this amount, a portion of wholemeal pasta, rice, couscous, high-fibre breakfast cereal or small baked potato is roughly equivalent to a slice of wholemeal bread and can help to increase your fibre intake. A typical day might start with wholemeal toast and/or porridge, or muesli with the addition of fresh or dried fruit. Opt for a baked potato with some broccoli, sweetcorn or baked beans for lunch; an apple, pear and banana for snacks and you have upped your intake of fibre. Not exactly difficult to achieve! The healthy target for fibre (NSP) is 20 grams per day for men and slightly less (16–18 grams) for women.

Fibre Facts

- A portion of carrots will give you 1.5 grams of fibre; a couple of sprigs of broccoli will give you 2.1 grams.
- All dried fruits are a good source of fibre but one fig will give you more than one prune, date or apricot.
- A medium-sized banana or kiwi fruit has 1.1 grams, and a medium-sized pear has 3.5 grams of fibre.
- Two small, round oatcakes yield 2 grams of fibre.
- A portion of frozen peas will give you 8 grams of fibre, a portion of canned peas will provide 4 grams.
- Baked beans, canned in tomato sauce, will provide 5 grams of fibre, and so will the same medium-sized portion of sweetcorn kernels.
- Choose a high-fibre breakfast cereal to start the day or as a mini meal. Check the nutrition label – at least 6 grams of fibre per 100 grams is good.

Table 1. How Much Fibre?

Most people do not include enough fibre (NSP) in their diet. The aim is to eat around 18 grams of NSP per day.

The foods listed below will each supply 5 grams of NSP

2 slices (large loaf, medium sliced) wholemeal bread
5 slices white bread
2 thick slices malt loaf
2 wholemeal fruit scones
5 cheese scones

2 tablespoons (1/3 small bowl) All Bran
Small serving (1/2 medium bowl) Bran Flakes

1 medium bowl of Fruit'n Fibre
5 medium bowls of Cornflakes or Special K
1½ large bowls of porridge
10 large bowls of Rice Krispies or Coco Pops
1 small bowl Sultana Bran, Shreddies
  or 1 Shredded Wheat
3 Weetabix

2 large bananas
3 large apples
2 small oranges
2 pears

4 dried apricots
2 large dried figs
8 stewed or ready to eat prunes

1 large bowl lentil soup or vegetable broth
6 bowls of tomato, chicken or oxtail soup

1 small portion peas
1½ servings of tinned sweetcorn
2 heaped teaspoons baked beans
4 tablespoons pea and potato curry
6 large tomatoes
3 large servings of cabbage
3 large pieces of steamed broccoli
4 medium-sized boiled potatoes, no skin

The F Word

Some high-fibre foods have had a hard time fighting against the image of the F word – flatulence! Kidney beans, baked beans, soya beans, peas and lentils are some of the worst offenders (one study found that eating baked beans increased the gas production in the intestines by 12 times!). This is because they contain raffinose and stachyose, two sugars which our digestive enzymes simply cannot break down. They are, however, broken down later in the large intestine by bacteria, which produce gas as a by-product of their leguminous meal. Horticulturists have had some success in developing beans with a low sugar content and therefore a lower flatulence factor. The trick is not to eat too many of them, too often, but ginger, peppermint tea and garlic as part of a meal are natural remedies and help to expel wind.

The Dangers of Dehydration

As you eat more fibre, it is important to increase your fluid intake as well. This enables the fibre to swell and increase in bulk. Fibre is not effective if it is not mixed with water and, anyway, it would be a real struggle to eat a bowl of All Bran or muesli without some form of fluid!

Whether they include fibre in their diet or not, most people simply don't drink enough – and then wonder why they get dehydration headaches! We live and work in air-conditioned or centrally-heated buildings where the air is recycled, and with each turn draws moisture out of the body. Water makes up the largest component in a human being. Men can be rather unflatteringly described as 65–75 per cent water (that's around 55 litres of water sloshing about). In comparison, women have a lower body water content (55–65 per cent) since they have less muscle tissue and a greater proportion of adipose tissue, and fat is a relatively 'dry' substance. We are constantly losing water via our lungs, in sweat and when we visit the toilet. This fluid needs to be replaced since both mental and physical performance is compromised by even mild dehydration. Aim for a daily intake of at least three litres of various fluids, including water (bottled or filtered if possible), fruit juices, herb and fruit teas, soup or milk.

Thirst is not a good indication of fluid needs. By the time the brain has been triggered and we feel thirsty, it is too late; you are already dehydrated. The best indication of your fluid needs is the colour of your urine; it should be a pale straw colour. If it is dark orange, then you need to drink more.

Endless cups of coffee to combat dehydration is not a good strategy. It may seem that you are replacing fluids, but caffeine is a diuretic and so promotes further fluid loss. As discussed in the next chapter, caffeine can also be a major energy drainer!

2

Caffeine – The Energy Drainer

Do you enjoy an occasional espresso with the after dinner mints, or do you make a more regular contribution to the 2.5 billion cups of coffee drunk each day? If so, it may be time to re-think your habit and discover that caffeine, the very substance you believed was keeping you going, is actually draining your mental energy!

It all began, so legend has it, many centuries ago when an Arabian goatherd noticed that his animals became particularly frisky after grazing on the red berries growing on nearby bushes. He told the monks who then collected the berries and made a brew which kept them awake during the long hours of prayer. Although the monks did not advertise the new beverage, the word was soon spread by visiting pilgrims travelling to Mecca. In sixteenth century Egypt it was declared illegal, because of its intoxicating effects, and the new coffee houses were burned.

Today, caffeine is the world's most popular stimulant. A total of 120,000 tons of it are consumed each year, equivalent to half a cup of coffee for every person on the planet. Although both tea and coffee contain caffeine, the concentration in tea is much less and tea also has some other redeeming qualities. Nevertheless, drinking some type of caffeinated drink is part of our culture and everyday life. We visit a friend and on goes the kettle, business meetings break for coffee, and in every corridor in every organization is a sophisticated coffee and tea making machine. And yet the caffeine intake is probably contributing to everyday stress. In the UK, 270,000 people take time off work every day because of stress-related illness; this means a cumulative cost in sick pay, lost production and the National Health Service bill of around £7 billion each year – and rising. Many of the largest and most successful companies are spending vast sums of money on stress management, team-building strategies and dealing with emotional issues. Marks and Spencer, Glaxo and Ford are three of many blue chip companies that provide 'employee assistance programmes'. Others are exploring all possible methods which might lead to increased productivity and performance from each individual. One of the answers is probably staring them in the face – from the bottom of their coffee cup! The caffeine intake of employees is no doubt a significant factor on work-related stress, especially where shift work is involved.

A vast amount of research has been carried out, mainly in the last five years, on the effects of caffeine on the mind and body. It is now generally agreed that caffeine can contribute to stress. This is unfortunate for the 140,000 travellers who pass through London's Gatwick airport each day, and have a fear of flying. In 1995, 1.4 million cups of coffee (equivalent to 5.2 tons of coffee beans) were served in an effort to calm them down! Caffeine is not technically classed as an addictive drug, but certainly many people depend upon it and suffer significant withdrawal symptoms if they go without their regular stimulant fix. They complain of a 'washed out' feeling, tiredness, headaches and general unwellness. These are exactly some of the sensations that anyone recovering from an operation would suffer. We are told that they are because of the after-effects of the anaesthetic, but a recent study has suggested that it is because of caffeine withdrawal. It is common practice to tell patients to avoid taking any drink containing caffeine both immediately before and after surgery.

Stimulating Research

There has been a phenomenal number of studies to investigate the health and so called energy-giving aspects of caffeine. One recent review on its effect on the central nervous system included 656 references! Caffeine has been linked with everything from causing heart disease and cancers to heartburn and birth defects. The links are tenuous – except if you live in Scandinavia where coffee drinking has a definite effect on blood cholesterol levels, causing them to rise. However, this is because of the way the drink is made, rather than a direct effect of caffeine itself. The coffee in Scandinavian countries is generally prepared by prolonged boiling of the coffee grounds in water, and then it is drunk without being filtered. Boiling the coffee is thought to release fatty acids from the bean which can raise blood cholesterol, one of the many risk factors for coronary heart disease.

Many other studies which have investigated the effects of instant coffee have concluded that there is no link between caffeine and raised blood cholesterol. Caffeine does, however, affect blood pressure and heart rate. Anyone with heart problems or who suffers from arrhythmias would be wise to avoid caffeine. Whilst there is general agreement that the risk of developing life-threatening diseases from drinking coffee is small, the effects of caffeine on how we feel, our energy levels and mood are much more dramatic.

The chemical name for caffeine is 1,3,7-trimethylxanthine. In its pure form it is a bitter-tasting fine white powder, looking rather like icing sugar. It is soluble in water so is easily absorbed into the bloodstream and rapidly reaches the brain where its most remarkable effects are felt. In general, a single dose of caffeine will appear in the bloodstream within 10 minutes of drinking it. It then reaches a peak concentration between 30 and 60 minutes after taking it, but absorption is much slower when the stomach is full. Experiments which measured the electrical activity of the brain have shown that the caffeine in just one or two cups of instant coffee dramatically changes the pattern of activity from a typical resting state to that of an alert, very awake person. It was found that repetitive tasks needing total concentration were done much better after a dose of caffeine. This led an American computer company to supply its employees with a caffeine-loaded soft drink called 'Jolt'. The drink was provided freely throughout the day to encourage maximum work output!

Caffeine has its effect on the brain by blocking the action of adenosine, another psychoactive chemical. It is a chemical which is found throughout the body and is an important regulator of energy metabolism. Adenosine is also involved in the transmission of electrical impulses along nerves. Having said all this, you would think that adenosine is a real live wire and an energizing substance; but it is not. If you inject adenosine, or any other substances that increases adenosine levels, into the body it has a calming effect. It lowers blood pressure, heart rate and body temperature, protects against seizures, slows down the motility of the digestive tract and generally balances the body's reaction to stress. In large amounts it can make you feel quite lethargic and sleepy. This is because adenosine can slow down the release of neurotransmitters – chemicals that carry messages from one nerve cell to another. To do this, the adenosine molecule must first bind to specific receptor sites on the cell surface. Caffeine has a molecular structure that is so similar to adenosine, that it can bind to the same receptor sites and block the action of adenosine. Without the calming and controlling effect of adenosine, nerve cells continue to fire – and fire more rapidly. As long as the caffeine molecules sit on the receptor sites, we are literally firing on all cylinders.

Caffeine also raises the levels of two key stress hormones, adrenalin and cortisol. These are the ones that are released when we get anxious, scared, angry or nervous; they produce the well-known jittery fight or flight feeling. Overall, caffeine not only increases the body's stress levels, but also blocks the action of adenosine, one of the body's de-stressing chemicals. No wonder we feel high and alert after every cup of coffee.

Caffeine will continue to have its effects as long as it remains in the bloodstream. In the meantime, enzymes in the liver work to break down the drug and remove it from the system. The half-life of caffeine – the amount of time it takes for the liver to metabolize half of the amount that has been taken in – varies a great deal between individuals. The usual half-life for an adult is between two to ten hours, with an average of around four hours. This huge variation explains why some people can drink large amounts of coffee without much effect, whilst others are jittery, anxious and simply cannot tolerate caffeine. Men and women tend to have similar rates of caffeine metabolism. Smoking stimulates the enzymes that metabolize caffeine, and smokers have a 50 per cent faster rate (half-life of three hours) compared with non-smokers. This means that smokers experience the effects of caffeine for a shorter time and possibly drink more to compensate. Other drugs, such as alcohol, reduce the rate of caffeine breakdown, and the oral contraceptive pill can more than triple the half-life of caffeine. Thus women on the pill tend to react strongly to a second dose of caffeine because there is still a large amount waiting to be metabolized.

Although there is individual variability in the reaction to caffeine, one thing is clear – people who drink a lot of coffee on a regular basis do develop a tolerance to it, meaning they need to drink more and more to get the same 'buzz'. In fact, once you get to this level, caffeine starts to have other less desirable effects on the body. In a sense you become over-stimulated; you are jittery, anxious, on edge all the time, nervous and sometimes visibly unsteady. Known as the 'coffee shakes' this is caused by caffeine disrupting the fine motor co-ordination within the nerves. These are also the symptoms that drive people to their first cup of the day.

A recent study showed clearly that overnight caffeine deprivation is enough to induce significant negative effects, including tiredness, headaches, depressed mood, anger and dejection. Once you have downed your first dose of caffeine, these feelings are relieved. This leads people to think that caffeine is making them feel better, but it is simply covering up the effects of too much and a tolerance to it. On top of this it adds to the overall stress of the body, so no wonder caffeine drinkers wake up in the morning feeling lousy. The feelings of withdrawal are an indication that a powerful, toxic chemical is being drained from your body.

The Benefits of Giving Up Caffeine

I found out from personal experience, the benefits of giving up the stimulant and not relying on caffeine to get me through each day. It all began a few years ago when a friend of mine came to me for advice, complaining that he was lacking in energy. He had just started a new job in which he wanted to do well, but each morning he would drag his 38-year-old body out of bed and then struggle through the rest of the day. Each day he would dash to the station to catch the early train to work and then sleep for the whole two-hour journey, thinking that he was tired because of his early start. When he arrived at the office, he would immediately reach for the coffee jar before he could even begin to think about doing anything else. 'I needed a cup of coffee to get me started and then I drink tea and coffee throughout the day.' He also ate chocolate bars, hoping that it would give him the quick energy boost that he needed. No matter what he did, he always felt tired, and with crucial meetings and presentations to give, each day was a real struggle. He wanted me to give him some new energy pill or vitaminized drink that would boost his system.

Once I'd had a look at the details of what he was eating, I decided not to put something into his diet to boost his energy levels, but to take a couple of things out. One of these was sugar, the other was caffeine. I also realized that I was drinking a lot of coffee so, four years ago, we both agreed to give up caffeine. It proved to be a challenge for us both, especially getting through the initial withdrawal symptoms. We suffered severe headaches, tension at the back of the neck and bad temper – it all felt rather like a dose of flu and lasted for about five days. But, oh was it worth it; we are now changed people! My friend no longer feels tired and has to buy two quality newspapers which he reads from cover to cover on the journey to work. He doesn't touch the coffee jar and no longer craves chocolate. He feels alive, really enjoys his work and is much more productive because he feels so well – even though he is still under a lot of pressure. I, too, feel different and much less tense without caffeine flooding my system every day. I have even more energy than I used to (which for a nutritionist is a good advert!) and I am calmer, even though I run my own consultancy business, write books and articles for magazines and newspapers, give seminars and lectures, design and run my own courses and do television and radio work! I enjoy the flavour of coffee, but if I drink it now I soon feel sluggish and develop a headache. I prefer to relish the aroma when I visit a coffee house, which is much more pleasant than the effects caffeine has on my system.

Although I was overjoyed at the benefits that two people found when they gave up caffeine, it got me thinking – I wonder if other people experience the same benefits. Plenty of studies have been done to examine the effects of caffeine on blood pressure or heart rate or kidney function, but no one as far as I was aware, had investigated the effects on personality and general mental performance. I had a contract with the Lifestyle Health Promotion programme which was run for the giant oil exploration and production company, Shell Expro UK. This involved travelling to a number of production platforms in the North Sea to give talks and seminars to the off-shore teams. Alcohol is banned off-shore – but an awful lot of coffee and other sources of caffeine are consumed instead. Here was an ideal opportunity to carry out a small research project on the effects of giving up (or cutting down), caffeine. It was a very simple study and involved filling in questionnaires. First, volunteers were asked questions relating to who they were, their work schedule, how much caffeine they consumed each day, and to give a self-assessed rating of their physical and mental state. They then agreed to take the 'Caffeine Challenge', which was to give up caffeine for a month. At the end of the four weeks, they were sent a second questionnaire, again asking them to rate and describe their mood and mental state. As the questionnaires came flooding in, it was clear that individuals working off-shore certainly did consume a large amount of caffeine (the average daily intake was 929 mg). Office workers based on-shore were also encouraged to take the 'Caffeine Challenge' and, with a coffee machine on every floor, they too heavily relied on the stimulant (average daily intake was 903 mg). A dose of 100 mg (the amount usually found in a single cup of coffee), will normally produce the stimulating effects we associate with the drug. An intake over 500 mg per day is considered high, and is the level at which many individuals begin to experience the downside of the stimulant's effects; moodiness, anxiety, fretfulness and tension.

I was amazed and surprised at the number of ways many of the 'guinea pigs' had benefited from cutting out caffeine or significantly reducing their intake. Several off-shore engineers reported that they no longer had headaches and could work much more productively as a team because they were no longer so tense and wound up. The safety officer was delighted when his tinnitus (buzzing, thumping, ringing sound in the ears) was cured. Mike, working in the helicopter flight control room, announced that he had tried to give up smoking every year for the past 16 years, but always caved in after a couple of weeks. Since giving up caffeine, he has gone for seven months without a cigarette. 'I always associated smoking with drinking coffee, but now I don't miss either!'

Paul worked as a computer programmer, which he enjoyed, but every weekend he suffered from headaches and felt generally depressed, tired and anxious. His wife objected to his grumpy moods, especially as they soon disappeared once he was back at work and away from her! Taking part in the 'Caffeine Challenge' highlighted the fact that he drank strong coffee continually throughout the day, which meant at weekends, when he hardly drank any, he was displaying withdrawal symptoms. Paul reckoned that changing his coffee drinking habits at work probably saved his marriage! It no doubt eased his overworked kidneys too. Caffeine is a diuretic, artificially stimulating the production of urine. Many of the 'Challenge' guinea pigs reported not having to visit the toilet so often (especially during the night), having cut down their caffeine intake! This has its own practical advantages, but it also means that the body retains more of the vital vitamins that are otherwise excreted with the increased flow of urine every day. Normally the kidneys are able to selectively excrete the toxic chemicals but retain other essential nutrients. In particular the B vitamins are lost when a lot of caffeine is taken. These play a crucial role in energy metabolism and so, with a high caffeine intake, the body is losing the very nutrients that are needed to produce energy. No wonder we feel tired, not only in the mind, but also the body!

Caffeine and Sleep

The highly subjective reports from individuals who noticed that they slept much more soundly after taking part in the 'Caffeine Challenge' confirm the results of a much more controlled experiment, on the effects of caffeine on sleep, carried out in Japan. Volunteers who took 150 mg of caffeine, then took an average of 126 minutes to get to sleep compared with 29 minutes for those who had not taken caffeine. The caffeine users slept for a total of 281 minutes in the laboratory compared with 444 minutes for the non-caffeine users. Recordings of the electrical activity of the brain showed that caffeine in all cases significantly altered normal sleep patterns, and many other similar studies have confirmed these findings. They also show that caffeine users are more easily aroused by sudden noises, they move about and are generally a lot less settled during sleep – and on waking report that they don't feel as though they have had a good night's sleep.

The sleeping body gives the impression of being totally switched off; it is not. This is dealt with further in the next chapter, but sleep is a time when transmitters and cells are recharged, the brain recovers from the stresses and strains of the day, and tissues are revitalized. Overall, it is as vital for subconscious activity as for physical passivity.

There are two types of sleep: dream sleep, also known as REM (Rapid Eye Movement) and deep sleep, or non-REM. Any growth or repair of the body occurs during deep sleep, but REM (which occurs towards the end of the sleep time) is for psychological repair. This is the time when the mind can unwind, and sort through information stacked away in our sub-conscious during the day.

This is the best time for coming up with solutions to challenges that you simply couldn't figure out during waking hours. Without adequate REM sleep we become fretful, irritable, tense and less able to concentrate. It is thought that caffeine may affect the quality of REM sleep, and so contribute to feelings of restlessness at a deeper level.

By now you should be convinced that giving up (or cutting down) on your caffeine intake is worth a try. At the very least you can only discover the benefits. A question I am often asked is: 'What do I drink instead?' Remember, it is important to drink at least three litres of fluid each day. When you give up coffee, you need to find a replacement beverage – which doesn't contain caffeine –some Colas and soft drinks contain caffeine and this is usually added as a flavouring and may be listed in the ingredients. Tables 2 and 3 give more details about the caffeine content of various drinks and foods.

Table 2. Caffeine-containing Drinks and Foods

Tea (all types of black tea). Green tea (served in Chinese restaurants) is low in caffeine.

Coffee (instant, mellow instant, espresso, cappuccino, Turkish, Continental blends, percolated and filter coffee).

Lucozade, Iron Bru and Cola soft drinks (NB: Diet versions of soft drinks contain much less sugar, but the same amount of caffeine).

Chocolate bars (dark chocolate contains four times as much caffeine as milk chocolate). The amount of chocolate in a serving of ice-cream, gateaux, or pudding is negligible in terms of the amount of caffeine it provides.

Anadin, Paracetamol tablets and powdered cold remedies (e.g. Lemsip) contain caffeine!

Caffeine Content of Various Beverages and Foods

(data from the Coffee Science Information Centre)

	Average amount (per 150 ml cup or as stated) mg	Range mg
Ground coffee	115	60–180
Instant coffee	65	30–120
Tea	40	20–60
Cocoa	4	2–20
Drinking chocolate	4	2–15

Decaffeinated coffee	4	2–4
Decaffeinated tea	3	2–4
Cola (330ml can)	40	30–40
Dark chocolate (100 g bar)	80	70–90
Milk chocolate (100 g bar)	20	4–60
Painkillers (two tablets)	60	30–130
Lucozade (330 ml can)	40	30–40

Table 3. Caffeine-free (or very low level) Drinks and Foods

Decaffeinated tea and coffee.
Green China tea.
Herbal teas (mint, chamomile, lemon verbena, fennel, rosehip).
Cocoa, drinking chocolate, chocolate Horlicks and all instant chocolate-containing drinks.
Fruit teas (Orange Dazzler, Apple Magic, Blackcurrant Bracer, Raspberry Rendezvous, Lemon and Lime).
Fruit juices (try concentrated apple juice diluted with hot water and add a few cloves).
Fruit squashes.
Lucozade Sport and other sports drinks (check the label).
Ribena (try it with hot water).
Fizzy fruit/soft drinks (Lilt, Tango, lemonade, ginger beer).
Mixers (ginger ale, bitter lemon, tonic water, etc.).
Caffeine-free Pepsi and Coke.
Milk.

The exact amount of caffeine in a cup of coffee or tea varies tremendously. The range for coffee is from 30–180 mg and for tea it is 20–60 mg. The wide variation is mainly because of the size of the cup, the quantity and quality of the coffee or tea leaf used and the method of brew. For example, filter coffee surprisingly contains more caffeine than percolated coffee which in turn contains more than instant. This is because in making filter coffee, although the water passes over the beans only once, nearly all of the caffeine is dissolved out of the more finely ground coffee. Repeatedly washing the coffee, as in the percolated method, only causes more of the other substances in the bean to go into solution. Although the actual content of caffeine in tea is greater than in coffee, on average, a cup of tea usually contains less. Caffeine is also released from tea leaves more slowly, especially if the leaves are in tea bags.

It is possible to cut down your caffeine intake quite dramatically simply by drinking tea instead of coffee. This is good news for everyone who really enjoys a good cup of tea, or who has to choose a drink when only tea or coffee are on offer. Green China tea is virtually caffeine free and is best drunk without milk. It has an unusual smokey flavour and is perhaps an acquired taste. So are many of the new herb and fruit teas which are storming onto the market as alternative caffeine-free drinks. In the past few years, sales of these in the UK have rocketed, and in 1996 we drank 1,397 million cups of herbal teas alone. This is a small brew compared with other European countries; 70 per cent of Germans and 50 per cent of French people drink herbal teas daily. Herb teas are made with the flowers, leaves and stems of all kinds of aromatic plants. Apart from being caffeine-free, their mild healing properties have been valued for centuries. If you want to experiment, try the following:

Chamomile – to calm your digestion and as a gentle sedative and relaxant.

Peppermint – to aid digestion and relieve flatulence.

Nettle – as a general tonic, but also to settle nerves.

Lime flowers – to relieve anxiety and nervous tension.

Ginger – an internal antiseptic and anti-inflammatory agent.

Elderflower – a general tonic and mild laxative.

Fruit teas are simply flavoured water. If you read the list of ingredients you will find that any fruit tea will always include hibiscus and rose hip. These give what the tea manufacturers call 'body'. Flavourings are then added to the basic mix to create anything from strawberry tea to more exotic blends such as 'Mango and Apple' or 'Passion fruit and Pear'. They are a good choice if you want a no-caffeine drink, and with all the varieties on the market, you won't get bored with the same flavour.

Coffee substitutes, which have never seen a coffee bean, are also available and popular on the Continent. They usually contain a mixture of roasted barley, chicory, figs, rye, wheat, dandelion root or acorns. Make sure to avoid the ones that contain guarana – a Brazilian herb and a source of caffeine!

What About Decaffeinated Tea and Coffee?

If you want to cut down on your caffeine intake, but still enjoy the flavour of coffee, then choose de-caff. Make sure that you check the label first because there are two methods used to decaffeinate the coffee beans; one is much healthier than the other.

Caffeine is removed from the coffee beans or tea leaves at the green stage, before roasting or fermentation, by 'washing' with water or a solvent. The solvent is either methyl chloride (the basis of paint stripper), or ethyl chloride (better known as a dry cleaning fluid!). These solvents can leave residues which are possibly as harmful as the caffeine they are removing. The other method, known as the Swiss Water Method, involves water, carbon dioxide and steam to remove the caffeine. It is more expensive but obviously does not create harmful residues. Both methods involve heat treatments which can destroy some of the coffee flavour components.

Most decaffeinated tea is made using the solvent extraction method, but you need to read the label to check which method has been used. If the label is vague about the method of decaffeination, it has probably been done using the solvent method!

The pure caffeine that is extracted is not wasted. It is ladled back into soft drinks and also many over-the-counter cold remedies and headache pills. So, if you suffer from a withdrawal headache as you cut down on your caffeine intake, remember not to reach for an alternative source in the form of a headache pill!

3

Synchronize Your Biological Rhythms

It's a familiar pattern. There are times during the day when you are firing on all cylinders – feeling particularly alive and focused, coping well with your work and shining at business meetings, or somehow coping with the demands of small children that would otherwise leave you frazzled. Yet there are other times – in the same day – when you find yourself making simple inexplicable errors, and unable to concentrate or think clearly. The period of fatigue and yawning that can descend around mid-afternoon is a common occurrence, but a couple of hours later we seem to have pepped up again and found a second wind. Most people believe that this spaced-out feeling results from the large meal they had for lunch. This is true to some extent – a full stomach does cause a diversion of blood supply to the intestine, which cuts back on the flow to the brain. But have you ever noticed that you don't get quite the same effect after a large breakfast? The mid-afternoon lethargy also occurs if you only have a small snack for lunch. So what's going on? What we eat is only partly to blame for the change in our mood and energy levels throughout the day; our mind and body activities are also ruled by natural cycles and rhythms.

Tune In to Your Biological Clock

Since the beginning of time, civilizations have set their routines and pace of life by the external cycles of the Sun and Moon. Only recently have we realized that we have our own internal clocks which also play a vital role in our everyday lives. Our bodies follow a pre-programmed sequence so that the essential functions of sleep, wakefulness, growth, repair and metabolism occur during the most appropriate times of day or night.

You may be familiar with the term circadian rhythm which refers to the biological cycle that occurs over 24 hours. Originally it was thought that our circadian rhythm was simply a daily alternation between being awake and asleep, but research now shows that there are other rhythms which have a powerful effect on how we feel and how efficiently we perform throughout the day. So, to maximize your everyday performance, you should tune in to your internal clock!

The exact site of the body clock in humans has yet to be determined, but in rats and other mammals it is located in two small groups of cells, one on either side of the brain, called the suprachiasmatic nuclei (SCN). The siting of the clock in this area is significant because the cells are part of a larger area known as the hypothalamus, a region of the brain that also controls body temperature, food and water intake, hormone secretion and sexual drive. When the SCN were removed, it was found that the rats' cycles of feeding, drinking and sexual activity were destroyed.

Wherever the clock is located in our bodies, there is no doubt that it is a sophisticated device, 'ticking' away and controlling what we feel – and when we feel it. The sleep/wake cycle is one of the body's most powerful rhythms that makes us feel alert during the day and sleepy at night. However, a

British study carried out at Manchester University suggests that our cycle does not exactly coincide with the planet's 24-hour day. Kept in a room with continuous artificial light, and none of the daily external cues as a guide, the bodies of the Manchester test group adjusted to a 25-hour cycle.

This happens to many of us at weekends. Without alarm clocks, deadlines and appointments, staying up late on Friday or spending half of Sunday in bed, our rhythms free run onto the natural 25-hour cycle. People who are particularly sensitive find themselves feeling sluggish with the 'Monday morning blues' as they report to work slightly 'jet-lagged'. People suffering from blindness caused by retinal disease often lose synchrony with their family, friends and colleagues as their daily rhythm free-runs on a 25-hour cycle.

Research has shown that there are distinct variations, ruled by the circadian rhythms, in our physical and mental abilities. This is because during each complete cycle, body temperature, urine production, levels of glucose, cholesterol and other substances all rise and fall; our mood mind and body are constantly changing throughout the day and night.

Putting it all together – a typical day would begin around 7 a.m. Having sunk to its lowest point some time between 4 a.m. and 6 a.m., our body temperature begins to rise rapidly. This affects our metabolism, which also starts to speed up because enzymes (controlling various chemical processes in the body) work faster when the temperature is higher. These in turn kick-start the release of the rousing hormone cortisol, and we reach our peak mental performance some time between 7 a.m. and 12 noon. This is the best time for tackling any problems – the boss or an important piece of work. After midday is not a good time for making decisions. Our body temperature starts to cool off again, levels of adrenalin and other hormones decrease, and mental ability generally gets put on the back-burner. This is when most people feel lethargic and notice a definite drop in efficiency.

People who work in Mediterranean countries have the right idea when they break off and have a siesta. It happens to coincide with the hottest part of the day – but it makes sense to synchronize with your body-cycles rather than fighting against them. After 3 p.m. our mental ability begins to pick up again and we can work well. From 4 p.m. to 7 p.m. we are at our physical peak thanks to a rise in levels of the hormones, noradrenalin and adrenalin (the new names for these are norepinephrine and epinephrine). These affect optimal nerve functioning and muscle co-ordination which helps manual workers to perform well, but this is the time to challenge for a game of squash or engage in some form of exercise. From 7 p.m. onwards, the body cools down along with the metabolic rate and levels of various hormones until we are back to our lowest ebb at 3 a.m. With this knowledge it is possible to schedule important business meetings or conference calls to take advantage of these peaks. As well as circadian rhythms, there are other cycles which may have a more immediate effect on our mood and overall health.

Tune In to Your Ultradian Rhythms

Sleep is an active, not a passive time and, as already mentioned, it is divided into periods of dream sleep known as REM (Rapid Eye Movement) and non-REM sleep. The shift between the two types has been found to occur every 90–120 minutes. As explained in Chapter 2, caffeine interferes with the REM phases of sleep which in turn has a profound effect on our mood, energy levels and performance.

New and exciting research has suggested that these 90–120 minute cycles continue when we are awake and also have a significant and deep effect on our performance, stress and energy levels. They are called ultradian rhythms, from ultra-dies meaning 'beyond' or many times per day. At the peak of your ultradian rhythm you are in a state of arousal which is perfect for learning or concentrating on difficult tasks. Your mind is clear, you are more alert and you can think and speak faster because your sensory and motor nerves are at their peak. In order to achieve this state, you need to have a good in-built recovery phase, which is where the troughs come in. This is when your mental and physical housekeeping occurs. Cells are re-vitalized and re-charged ready to move up to the next peak, but at this time your outward performance is reduced. You feel drowsy, and cannot think straight, which is an ideal time for ploughing through some of the more mundane tasks – filing, easy reading, routine phone calls.

Ultradian rhythms effectively mean that our memory, creativity, mental concentration and physical performance rise and fall in cycles lasting 90–120 minutes. This implies that we can't expect to be firing on all cylinders for longer than a couple of hours at a time. Nevertheless, the demands of the day or our work schedules dictate that we strive for maximum performance for hours on end – which means ignoring the signs that we have reached a trough in one of our ultradian cycles.

Think about how you feel in conferences and business meetings that go on for longer than 90 minutes, or simply when working at your desk for extended periods. After a while, no matter how engaging the speaker, meeting or work, we reach a stage when we feel lethargic, our concentration lapses and our mind begins to wander. We inwardly chastise ourselves and persist in trying to plough through the troughs to bring ourselves back to peak concentration. More commonly we reach for a stimulant, in the form of a cup of coffee or a cigarette, to boost us back up to our maximum. The danger with this approach is that you deprive your body of the rejuvenation period needed for the next peak. In his book *The 20 Minute Break*, Ernest Rossi explores the power of these ultradian rhythms and concludes that 'maximum performance rests on this simple dictum: peak your peaks and trough your troughs'.

He goes on to explain: 'Peaks are good for outer performance; troughs are good for inner healing and inspiration. If you do not take advantage of the highs and lows, you disrupt your natural rhythm and fall into what is termed low-amplitude dysrhythmia. The lack of ultradian restoration leaves you with a deficit, so that you don't have the energy to carry yourself forward to the next natural peak. Performance mediocrity can result.'

When you become aware of the signals that you are entering a trough, the solution is simple – forget the coffee and nicotine stimulants and give yourself permission to relax and let your mind re-charge. Taking a breather is one of the most energizing things you can do! Stephen Hawking, one of the world's most creative astrophysicists, organizes his work day into a series of 90 to 120 minute periods of intense work with rest breaks in between. Ideally these should be 15–20 minutes of recovery time, but in a hectic day this is simply not always possible. When 'time is short and the water's rising', even allowing a small distraction – such as doodling, staring out of the window or reading the paper – can bring some benefit.

Those who try to keep going at all costs are taking the quickest route to a burnout. The only way to get through a hectic schedule is to build in regular recovery time. Top class and Olympic athletes used to think that success was built on intense training and running as many miles in a week as possible but, without sufficient recovery time, the athlete starts the session feeling weak and tired – hardly the best platform for an effective work-out. This philosophy has been radically changed, with positive results, by emphasizing the quality of training instead of the quantity.

'Few people do business well who do nothing else.'
– Lord Chesterfield

Take a Breather!

Simply removing yourself from your work site can have a calming effect. Taking a few deep breaths is also an excellent way to enhance the benefits of the short break and reduce stress by channelling new energy into your system.

We take breathing for granted. We tend to think that because it is something we do all the time, we know how to do it – but, often, we don't. Most of us breathe too cautiously, taking in only a tumblerful of air when we could benefit from taking in at least three times that amount. The lungs are made up of around 700 million air sacs. If our breathing is too shallow, we don't fully expel all the stale gases and pollution in the lower lungs. You cannot overdose on good deep breathing; the more oxygen you take in the more effectively you can energize your mind and body. Many of the Buddhist and Chinese healing rituals are based on deep breathing as a means of re-charging the vital life force of the body. There is a yoga proverb which says, 'Life is in the breath. Therefore he who only half-breathes, half-lives.'

When we are stressed or overworked, we tend to hold our breath. Sitting cramped over a desk for hours in a stuffy office is a sure way of reducing to a minimum the flow of oxygen to your cells. Although the brain weighs a fraction of our total body weight, it demands 25 per cent of the oxygen we take in. Fresh air can mean a fresh perspective and renewed energy. Just a couple of minutes of deep breathing several times each day will help.

There are many techniques for this but the basic rules are simple. Breathe as deeply as possible, taking air into the abdominal area and not just the upper chest. Begin by finding a comfortable position; stand up, move away from your desk, or lie down. Take several long, deep slow breaths, bringing air in through your nose rather than your mouth. As you do this, be aware of your abdomen and then your lungs filling almost completely with new air. Let your rib cage expand and your abdomen relax to make room for the oxygen. Hold your breath for five seconds and then slowly let the air out through your mouth. Exhale from the abdomen first. Feel your lungs collapsing and let your shoulders drop and relax as you let the air escape. If you do this with your eyes closed, imagine all the tightness and tension flowing from your body as you breathe out. Simply controlling your breathing like this is a simple way to reduce stress and re-oxygenate your body, whilst allowing inner healing to take place. If you can only manage to take one recharging break in a day, opt for mid-afternoon. Remember the mind and breath are closely connected. By controlling your breathing and making it very slow, you are calming down the noise of your mind.

Exercise – At Your Desk

Given half a chance we all tend to slouch when sitting for hours in a meeting or in front of a computer screen. Our shoulders become rounded, and we slump forward, which effectively upsets the way the spine is designed to carry the body's weight. By crowding the heart, lungs and stomach and the many organs needing, and expecting to be provided with plenty of space, it hampers their function. No wonder we feel sluggish and fatigued! Try these simple exercises to stimulate your circulation, release tension and ease any aches and stiffness.

Shoulder Shrugs

Stand away from your desk. Slowly raise your shoulders towards your ears as you breath in. Breath out and release. Repeat five times, then rotate your shoulders backwards and forwards five times.

Neck Rolls

With your body weight equally balanced on both feet, gently drop your chin to your chest, move your head to one side, come back down to the middle, then move your head to the other side. Do this a few times in each direction.

Back Relaxers

Stand firmly and raise your arms up as far as possible, keeping them close to your ears. Grasp your hands and push your palms up to the ceiling. Hold the stretch for five seconds and repeat twice more. Then grasp your hands behind your back, locking your fingers together. Keeping your back upright and straight, gently push your shoulders back as you raise your locked hands upwards as far as is comfortably possible. Hold for five seconds and repeat twice more.

Make these exercises part of your work day routine and they will help you to walk tall! Body language is important in all circumstances, but particularly so in business when gaining a person's confidence quickly is critical. A relaxed but confident posture conveys self-assurance and honesty. It encourages others to trust you and to take you seriously in any negotiations.

Massage Your Right Brain

When you are buried in work or are stuck for inspiration and ideas in a meeting, head massage can stimulate your creative right brain activity. The sense of touch must have preceded language by a long way and was probably the very earliest means of saying 'hello'. There is, therefore, a subtle creative right brain component in massage, and simply using fingertips to rub your scalp will have a soothing effect. The benefits, however subtle or small, will also travel around the body gently energizing and stimulating the immune system. Exactly how this works is difficult to explain. No scientist in a white coat has even measured the channels of energy, known as meridians, that are believed to flow through the body. Many of the healing therapies (including reflexology, acupuncture and shiatsu massage) are based on restoring health by unblocking the channels so that the body's energy can flow freely once more.

On-site massage is a service now offered by qualified therapists who regularly visit offices and give 20-minute treatments to employees, fully clothed and seated at their desks. The techniques are specifically designed to alleviate the tension resulting from working at a computer screen. On-site massage is a powerful preventive measure against repetitive strain injury (RSI) – and, incidentally, it is also very enjoyable!

Mid-Afternoon Low – Go With the Flow

The low that most of us feel at around 3 or 4 p.m. is because the natural low in our circadian rhythm coincides with a trough in one of the shorter ultradian ones. At this point, most of us find it easier to give in and let the natural recuperation occur. Top business executives, with an office of their own, can shut the door and hold all calls, but those on the 'shop floor' have less opportunity for a secluded session of inner healing. It is a shame that nodding off at one's desk is seen as a sign of inefficiency and weakness. The productivity of any company would be greatly enhanced if they entered into a mutually beneficial contract with its employees allowing them to get the job done by embracing the ultradian principles. The head of a private research laboratory has done just that. Dr Candice Pert encourages her co-workers to spend time in the quiet, solitary 'Zen' room whenever they need a restorative break. With this approach, it may not be a coincidence that this laboratory is at the forefront of some of the world's latest research into AIDS, psychobiology and brain biochemistry.

The Value of Sleep

Just as recovery during the day is important, sleep is the ultimate re-charger. Four hundred years ago Shakespeare wrote in *The Tempest*: 'We are such stuff as dreams are made on, and our little life is rounded with a sleep.'

His words are proving to be true. Not long ago sleep was considered to be something of a luxury, something that in our modern hectic world we could almost do without. After all, if Margaret Thatcher could manage on four hours each night, so could we! In fact, new research has confirmed what we always suspected, that a lack of sleep not only frays your temper but is bad for your health. According to the Sleep Disorders Clinic at St Georges Hospital Medical School in London, the Mrs Thatchers of this world are few and far between. Although the amount of sleep that we need each night lessens as we get older, we are genetically programmed to sleep a certain number of hours each night. For most people this is six to eight hours, with only 10 per cent of the population needing less. The problems start when we try to scrape by on a lot less and end up suffering from poor concentration and constant, low grade fatigue.

The message is, do not underestimate the potency of sleep to rejuvenate and energize your mind and body – as any one who is plagued by interrupted nights will testify! Working parents with young children are likely to have the worst of it. A clean nappy at 2 a.m. and a bottle at 4 a.m., only to get up at 6 a.m. to put on a business suit, load up the washing machine and be on the 8 a.m. train. It may be a passing phase, they try to reassure themselves, but the effects of stunted sleep take their toll on relationships, work, and health. So how do you know how much sleep you need? The answer is based on common sense; if you feel that you need to get more, then you probably do. Another test is how well you feel during the day. Do you find yourself sleeping on the bus, on the train, dozing off at your desk, during management meetings or even in the office toilets?

Active Re-charging

Research at the University of Toronto's Centre for Sleep and Chronobiology has revealed that sleep serves many purposes. Adequate sleep can help you fight diseases, delay the ageing process and even lose weight. Experiments have shown that the immune system is repaired and even bolstered during sleep. Blood samples taken during sleep revealed a surge in white blood cells which are an important part of the body's immune defence system. Several studies have shown that tired bodies are more likely to pick up bugs and infections because sleep loss disrupts this important immune system regeneration process. Night shift workers contract more infectious diseases than any other group, and hospital patients who have to be woken for treatment during the night, recover more quickly when they return home for a good sleep!

When our sleep patterns are disrupted, so are our other basic biological rhythms. It is easy to imagine that waves of contractions down the length of our digestive system are stimulated after a meal, but this peristalsis continues throughout the night. About four hours after the last meal of the day at the beginning of sleep, a slow wave starts in the stomach, and for the next 90 to 120 minutes continues down the small intestine and the large bowel. All night long these cycles of gentle contractions occur to keep the contents of the gut churning and moving, producing faeces ready to be expelled in the morning. It is significant that these rhythms last for 90 to 120 minutes as this is the interval between sleep stages in the brain. Dream sleep, or REM, should not be considered a lighter version to the deep or non-REM sleep, it is just different. Both are needed for complete rejuvenation of mind and body. REM sleep is when important psychological repair takes place and a chance for your mind to unload, unwind and sort through all the information and events of the day. Non-REM sleep is when agents of the body's repair kit are produced – including the churning cycles in the gut. It may be that non-REM sleep is essential for a healthy bowel, and perhaps some intestinal and digestive disorders stem from poor sleep patterns.

There is plenty of evidence to show that disrupted sleep can affect our appetite – we either lose it altogether or find that we are eating more because we are tired. The exact mechanism for this effect has not been confirmed, but during sleep the brain and the digestive system release several substances, including cytokines, Interleukin–1 and tumour necrosis factor. These have specific functions but are also thought to act as appetite suppressors. A simpler explanation is that when we are tired we comfort eat and turn to food to make us feel better. Exhausted people are much more likely to turn to low-nutrient-density fast foods and sugary snacks in the hope of getting a quick energy fix. A study in the USA confirmed that fatigue was at least one of the factors in overeating amongst a group of hospital nurses. In a survey across the country, 99 per cent of those working on night shift gained weight. From my own experience of working on offshore oil and gas platforms, comfort eating through boredom is very common – as the number of overweight night shift teams will confirm!

It is not laziness, but a pre-programmed biological system that drives us under the covers; our sleep/wake cycle is carefully programmed. It responds to the production of the hormone melatonin, often described as 'chemical sleep'. During darkness, the pineal gland in the brain releases a surge of melatonin into the bloodstream which causes our heart rate and digestion to slow, our blood pressure to drop and our minds to become less alert. When light hits the gland, this results in an almost immediate shut-down of melatonin and the body wakes up. This is why the hormone is so important – it establishes the basic rhythm of life for every organ, tissue and cell within the body.

When the natural sleep/wake cycles are disrupted, either by changing to working a night shift or flying to a different time zone, we certainly feel the effects. In fact, most night-shift workers are suffering from mild jet lag every time they clock on to a new shift. Unlike going over a hump back bridge and momentarily leaving your stomach behind, crossing time zones or working night shifts knocks the body's circadian rhythm for six. International business people are expected to be immune to this and to arrive ready to close a deal or make important decisions at times when, back home, they would normally be in their pyjamas!

The thousands of people who work during the night, particularly in high stress jobs where safety is at stake (airline crews, offshore drilling teams, surgeons, long distance lorry drivers), are regularly 'out of synch' with their body rhythms. Scientists working at the UK's Medical Research Council have shown a direct link between working on a night shift and increased accident rates. A huge amount of research on fatigue-related accidents also confirms that the majority of traffic accidents involving only one vehicle are more common during the early hours of the morning because of people falling asleep at the wheel. This is also the time when the world's most catastrophic accidents (Chernobyl, Three Mile Island and the Union Carbide explosion in Bhopal, India) occurred.

Such is the power of our biological clocks, and we should live by them, but unfortunately today's lifestyle often demands that we push ourselves beyond their limits. In overriding our body's signals to slow down, our natural rhythms become scrambled and our mood, energy levels and efficiency plummet as fatigue and stress set in. There are, though, ways to minimize the effects of disrupted cycles other than by tuning into your cycles and taking regular breaks.

How to Beat Jet Lag

Part of the problem with long-haul travel is dehydration. Travelling in an air-conditioned aircraft at altitude generally means being cooped up in an environment with only 5 per cent humidity. Re-hydrating the bodies inside the plane is a lot easier than re-humidifying the air to more comfortable levels (35 per cent). This would require 200 litres per hour on a 747, which mounts up to 2 tons of water on a 10 hour flight! The common sense remedy is to drink more and to do it more often. Sticking to fruit juices and water will promote rehydration – coffee, tea or alcohol are diuretics and will only serve to dehydrate you even more.

Fruit juices and tomato juice are also good sources of potassium. A long-haul journey is rather like a mini space flight – without the weightlessness. The body is confined with limited opportunity for exercise. Research at the Johnson Space Centre has shown that the immobility of overseas flights leads to the excretion of two vital minerals, sodium and potassium. These are important for optimal muscle and nerve performance and their loss accounts for the lethargy and muscle weakness that weary travellers often experience when they reach their destination. Taking as much 'exercise' during the flight (such as stretching, clenching and relaxing of muscles) and plenty of fruit and vegetable juices will help to preserve potassium levels.

The extent of the jet lag depends largely on the direction of travel. It is easier to move your body clock forwards than it is to move it backwards. This is why it is better to design shift-work patterns in a forward direction (e.g. night shift to morning shift to afternoon shift). The same applies to flying; it is easier to overcome jet lag when flying from east to west and adding a few more hours to the day than vice versa. When travelling from west to east, time is lost and it has been suggested that adaptation occurs at least 50 per cent slower. But what can be done to speed up the adaptation process?

Over the last few years melatonin supplements have been described as the miracle hormone, and the main benefit of these supplements lies in their ability to help in sleeping and in overcoming jet lag. Research (using over

500 mainly long-haul travellers) by Professor Josephine Arendt, Britain's leading expert on melatonin, at the University of Surrey showed positive results. The supplement's main benefits are the improvement of sleep and faster adaptation of the body's natural daily rhythms after arriving in a new time zone. Subjects flying across the Atlantic with a nine-hour time difference took a melatonin dose on the day of the journey and another on the evening of the day after they arrived. This had the effect of re-setting the body clock by two hours per dose. Instead of feeling washed-out for nine days, they got over the effects of travel in about three. Melatonin tablets can be freely purchased in the US and are currently selling faster than vitamin C. Melatonin was recently banned from sale in UK health food shops since it is classed as an unlicensed medicine and is only available on prescription.

Another time-honoured approach to beating jet lag (and a sign of an experienced long-distance traveller) is to re-set your watch to the new time as soon as you board the plane. Your mind then helps your body to speed up the adaptation process, and you eat when it is time to eat in the new time zone, even if it is way out in terms of the rhythms that you left behind.

To encourage sleep, choose starchy carbohydrate foods (bread, potatoes, soup, fresh and dried fruits, rice, pasta) with as little protein food as possible. This will encourage the production of serotonin (more of this in the next chapter) – the soothing, calming neurotransmitter that will help you sleep, even though the rest of your systems are a little further behind. It is best to resist the temptation to use alcohol to help you sleep. Although it may help you to relax and fall asleep, alcohol is a narcotic, numbing your brain and disrupting normal sleep patterns.

Have a Good Sleep

A third of our lives is spent sleeping – in an ideal world! Some of us are plagued by insomnia, and in 1996, 15 million prescriptions for sleeping pills were written for an estimated 1.5 million people in the UK. Although they may be safe and effective they should not be seen as a long term solution. A little time spent on working out the reasons why you can't sleep is a more productive approach. Nagging worries and stress are the most persistent enemies of a good night's sleep and there are several ways to overcome these. If you are a worrier then have a pen and paper handy by the bed so that vital thoughts can be scribbled down there and then. This relieves your sub-conscious mind of the anxiety of remembering until morning. The main trick is learning to relax. A hot bath and a warm drink (made with milk not an alcoholic tipple) will help. If you appreciate a good old-fashioned lullaby, there are plenty of relaxation tapes on the market specially devised to take over from where mother left off! These can be self-hypnosis tapes, but the soothing sounds of Bach, Schubert or Tchaikovsky are a blissful way to drift off. Most machines switch off automatically – but choose one that doesn't undo all the good work by making a loud clunk at the end!

4

Sugar, Food and Mood

To get us through the lows of the day, we reach for a bar of chocolate, or some other sweet snack. After all, sugar gives us energy – doesn't it? In some situations, particularly during exercise, it does; but mostly it actually contributes to that sleepy afternoon drowsiness that makes you sluggish. The annual UK National Food Statistics show that as a nation we consume an enormous amount of sugar, but by understanding the metabolism of sugar, you will see how, like caffeine, it can be an incredible drain on your energy.

Sugar Highs and Energy Lows

Let's get one thing straight, there is nothing wrong with foods that are naturally rich in sugar. Human beings love a sweet taste. Watch the expression on a young baby's face when it is given sugary water compared with the grimace it gives when something is bitter, and it is clear that from a very early age we know what we like! The in-built desire for sweetness goes way back to primitive times when our ancestors had to scrounge around for food and eat roots, shoots and berries. The only way to decide if a food was poisonous was by its taste. If it was sweet, chances were it would be harmless and safe to eat. Even today, nothing designed by nature, which is poisonous, is sweet.

Sugar is a form of carbohydrate and there are several different sugars: lactose is found in milk; fructose and glucose in fruits and honey. Sucrose occurs naturally in sugar beet and sugar cane, but the refined white sugar that sits in a sugar bowl is 99.9 per cent sucrose and is a highly processed product. During refining, all of the B vitamins and valuable trace minerals, such as calcium, iron, potassium and magnesium, are lost – leaving only Calories. It is these 'empty Calories' that are added in vast quantities to many of the foods consumed today. Food manufacturers have essentially cheated nature – which has always been perfectly capable of providing foods to satisfy our naturally sweet tooth.

In 1972, John Yudkin, Emeritus Professor of Nutrition at London University, wrote a book called *Pure, White And Deadly*. In it he examined the link between sucrose in the diet and health – the deadly aspect in the title refers to the negative effect that large amounts of sugar have on our metabolism and energy levels. It is no wonder that we suffer from fatigue, headaches, diabetes, migraines, constipation and high blood-pressure (as well as all of the life-threatening diseases) when you consider how much stress the food that we eat adds to our already hectic and stressed lives.

The day begins, as always, with the alarm clock which jolts you from a deep sleep to a gibbering wreck as you remember the series of deadlines stacked up for the day ahead. You head for the kitchen to grab something called breakfast. On automatic, you reach for the coffee jar and the box of sugar-coated cereal. This is followed by two slices of white bread, toasted and smeared with marmalade, and crammed into your mouth as you scan the paper, shove clothes into the washing machine or organize the children. Your day has begun – and it is likely to continue along the same pattern of reaching for a mouthful of something sweet to get a quick energy fix.

Foods with added sugar are concentrated and contain sucrose in unnaturally large amounts. A bowl of sugary breakfast cereal, your favourite chocolate bar, a couple of scoops of ice-cream, a piece of cake, a doughnut, a few biscuits – it is only a snack to you but to your digestive system it is the metabolic equivalent of a left hook from Mike Tyson. Suddenly your gut is hit with a cascade of sugar to absorb, and immediately your bloodstream is awash with glucose.

The way the body works is largely a matter of keeping the status quo. There are hormones which act as a network of sensors and controls to maintain a constant supply of glucose to the tissues and organs within the body. If anything causes a drop in blood glucose below normal, the hormone glucagon will be released which stimulates the breakdown of glycogen in the liver, which releases more sugar into the bloodstream. If the supply of glycogen gets low, a 'hungry' signal is sent to the brain. If the level of glucose in the blood rises above normal, then another hormone, insulin, is released which promptly causes the excess to be removed from the bloodstream (and stored in the liver and muscles as glycogen) until equilibrium is reached once more.

The problem with concentrated sugary foods (that most of us rely on to give us energy) is the flood of glucose into the bloodstream after we have eaten them. The level of glucose shoots up, rising too high, too quickly. This initiates a rapid response from insulin, but because of the large amount of glucose to deal with, too much insulin is released. This means that the sudden rise in blood glucose (known as hyperglycaemia) is followed by a dramatic fall (hypoglycaemia). Whilst your blood sugar is rising, you feel fine and 'energized', but this doesn't last very long. Within an hour of eating your sugary snack, your blood sugar comes crashing down – and you feel lousy. The symptoms of hypoglycaemia are dizziness, blurred vision, headaches, generally feeling weak and shaky. This is when you reach for another sugar fix, and the cycle of peaks and troughs continues throughout the day as you work at your desk and try to concentrate. How can you expect to work well when your blood glucose level behaves like a roller coaster that, when it hits rock bottom, saps your system and makes you addicted to the next energy surge?

Be a Nibbler, Not a Gorger

For peak mental performance you need a constant supply of fuel. Although the brain can only use glucose as a source of energy, eating concentrated sugary foods is not the answer. These cause sudden changes in brain sugar levels, and when the level is high you feel hyperactive. But what goes up, must come down, and pretty soon you feel sluggish and lethargic. It should be noted that this pattern applies to when we are physically inactive – sitting reading, writing, studying, or driving. A very different pattern of glucose metabolism occurs during exercise, when sugar then becomes a very useful source of energy.

There is normally the equivalent of one teaspoon of glucose circulating in your bloodstream, and a can of Cola drink, for instance, contains nine teaspoons of sugar. With this amount rushing into your resting system, no wonder the control mechanism goes haywire! Table 4 shows just how much sugar there is in other everyday, highly processed foods.

Table 4. Sugar Content of Some Foods

The recommended health target is to reduce sugar consumption to 1 lb (450 g) per person per week. This is equivalent to 12 teaspoons of sugar per day, from all sources!

Because of the amount of sugar added to foods, and hidden even in so called 'savoury' foods it is easy to exceed this recommended level.

Food	Teaspoons of Sugar
2 scoops of ice-cream	7
Individual pot of fruit yogurt	4
Bowl of cornflakes	1
Bowl of frosted breakfast cereal	4
1 cup of fizzy lemonade	4
1 small individual fruit pie	6
Small can of soup	1
Mars Bar	8
1 small jam doughnut	5
1 small (50 g) bar of milk chocolate	6
1 small Danish pastry	9
2 chocolate digestive biscuits	5
1 teaspoon of jam/marmalade	3
1 teaspoon of sweet pickle/chutney	3

Before you hold up your hands in horror and cry 'but I love sweet things, I don't want to give them up!', the answer is that you will not have to. There are plenty of wonderful foods which are naturally sweet and contain a much more diluted level of sugars which your metabolism can deal with more effectively and which don't result in energy highs and lows.

Table 5. Foods with Natural Sugar

(Compare the amount of sugar in these with those with added sugar in Table 4.)

Fruit	Natural Sugars (equivalent in teaspoons)
1 large orange	3
25 grapes	3
1 medium-sized banana	3
1 large apple	1
3 large plums	3
1 large peach or nectarine	1.5
1 large whole grapefruit	1
16 strawberries	2
11 cubes fresh pineapple	3
1 medium-sized pear	2
1 large whole Cantaloup melon	5
3 large fresh apricots	1.5
20 blackberries or raspberries	1.5
12 cherries	2

Think of all the fruits that are available and you have an endless choice of sweet-tasting, energizing snacks. Studies comparing the effects of eating little and often, against two or three large meals have consistently shown that performance, concentration, mood and overall health is better as a result of small frequent eating. This is how our jungle ancestors used to eat, snacking on fruits and berries throughout the day – and the same pattern of eating fits in well with our modern style of living where we want to eat on the move. Use fresh fruit as a snack – it is easy to eat and the perfect portable energizer. Aim to eat three or four pieces a day in between mini meals.

Here's how you can fit fruit into a hectic day:

Even-keel breakfast
High fibre cereal with chopped banana, skimmed or semi-skimmed milk, lemon tea.

Mid-morning laid back elevenses
Wholemeal sultana scone with fruit spread, honey or sugar-free jam. Herb or fruit tea.

Re-vitalizing lunch
Flaked tuna, veggies, green salad with lemon juice and Balsamic vinegar dressing or olive oil vinaigrette, fresh fruit salad.

Afternoon pick-me-ups
Apple, pear, orange or small bunch of grapes
OR
Thick sticks of cucumber and celery with thin sticks of cheese.

Wind-down dinner
Large bowl of vegetable or lentil soup with wholemeal crusty bread.
Chicken or cashew nut stir fry and baked potato.
Oaty apricot fruit crumble with Greek yogurt.

Sleep time snack
Banana and chamomile tea.

A piece of fresh fruit not only provides sugars, but comes with a package of vitamins and minerals and some fibre. The main type of sugar in fruit is fructose, which poses much less of a metabolic shock than other sugars. Fructose is absorbed and metabolized differently from the sucrose that is added to manufactured, highly processed sweet foods. Each molecule of fructose has to be gently 'escorted' across the gut wall and into the bloodstream via a process known as 'active transport', resulting in a slower absorption rate than with sucrose – which floods quickly through the intestine wall by simple diffusion. Once into the bloodstream, fructose, unlike sucrose, does not cause a rapid rise in insulin. Instead, fructose is taken to the liver and converted to glucose – which is then released slowly to maintain a sustained level of energy in the bloodstream.

So, eating more fruit is the answer. It not only provides the sweet taste that every human being enjoys, but its fructose content gives the energy highs without the lows. There are plenty of other reasons to eat more fruit each day (see Chapter 7). If you have a particularly sweet tooth, dried fruits – apricots, dates, figs, prunes, raisins and sultanas – are perfect to nibble on or to add to muesli, muffins, fruit or malt loaf as a sweetening agent. Leave out some of the added sugar in the recipe and use more dried fruit instead. Honey, the main sugar of which is also fructose, is another good sweetener. Not all sugars have the same level of sweetness, however. Lactose, the sugar found in milk, hardly tastes sweet at all.

Craving for Sugar

What if you really have an intense, seemingly uncontrollable, craving for sweet things. You regularly 'need' several bars of chocolate each day, and when you set out to nibble on a few biscuits – you end up eating the whole packet! A significant number of people find that this pattern of eating occurs during the long, cold, dark winter months. Many women find that it happens every month! Their healthy food choices and well-controlled appetite evaporates as pre-menstrual tension sets in! So what causes these food cravings?

Food and Mood

Biologists have believed for a long time that animals seek out and eat foods they not only find palatable, but which provide the nutrients that they particularly need. These needs seem to apply not only to the body, but the mind as well. New research suggests that food has a rapid effect on alertness and energy levels, memory and concentration and can even help to reduce depression. To what extent the foods we eat can affect our mood and mental performance is being studied by Dr Rogers, head of psychobiology at the Institute of Food Research in the south of England, and only one of a small number of British scientists exploring this field. The secret lies in the interaction of carbohydrates, proteins and fats from the foods that we eat throughout the day, and the theory is that, for most people, carbohydrates produce a calming and soothing effect, whilst proteins make us more alert.

The human brain is an incredible and complex organ. It has 100 billion nerve cells, and each cell can connect up with 10,000 others to create a wiring circuit which makes the most sophisticated computer look amateurish. Every sensation and thought that we have comes via an electrical impulse passing along nerve cells to the brain. The electrical charge is carried from one cell to another by neurotransmitters. Two of them, dopamine and serotonin, are especially concerned with pathways which generate a feel-good factor and help to maintain an overall sense of well-being.

Serotonin is a brain chemical which not only affects our mood but our appetite as well. We need optimum levels of serotonin to keep us on an even keel and make us feel good. The low mood in depression – the persistent feeling of sadness, emptiness, loss, dread and a lack of interest in life – is associated with decreased levels of serotonin. The reason why we crave sugary and highly refined carbohydrate foods is that they rapidly restore brain serotonin levels, which in turn make us feel good!

The question is, though, why are our serotonin levels low in the first place? One answer is that we don't eat enough carbohydrate in our diets to maintain optimum serotonin throughout the day. Most of the carbohydrate that we do eat is as highly processed starch or in the form of refined sugar – giving the highs and lows described earlier. Our serotonin levels follow this pattern, and when it drops to rock bottom, we know about it. We feel grumpy, low, depressed, moody, sad and generally sorry for ourselves. These are some of the symptoms experienced by women who suffer from PMT. The monthly cycle is controlled by fluctuating hormone levels, and at the end of the cycle there is a massive drop in levels of the hormone progesterone. This is accompanied by a dramatic fall in serotonin levels – which is why women tend to crave chocolate and other sweet foods at this time. We think we need a treat, so we reach for a sugary bun, a cake, some biscuits or a slab of chocolate. What we really need is a rapid boost of serotonin, which the sugar, indirectly, will provide.

An alternative, and more energizing approach is to encourage an optimum level of serotonin in the brain throughout the day. This can be achieved (and is the secret to beating those cravings) by eating much more of the starchy, unrefined carbohydrate foods – porridge, wholemeal bread, rice and pasta dishes, vegetable stir-fries, baked potatoes, corn on the cob, home made lentil, bean or vegetable soups.

Other foods have been found to contain a natural supply of pre-formed serotonin (see Table 6), which acts as a natural appetite supressant. Serotonin absorbed directly from foods does not pass across the blood-brain barrier, but binds onto receptor sites in the stomach which then send signals to the brain to suppress appetite. Serotonin-containing foods can, therefore, influence the amount of food you eat by registering 'fullness' via signals to the brain which tell us to stop eating!

Table 6. Foods Containing Serotonin

Avocado	Papaya/paw paw
Dates	Passion fruit
Banana	Plantain
Blue/red plums (not green)	Pineapple
Aubergine/eggplant	Tomato

Foods which provide carbohydrate are, therefore, the ideal foods for calming the brain and relieving stress and anxiety. If you are already well in control, they could make you feel drowsy, and certainly contribute to that mid-afternoon sleepy feeling which is largely dictated by our circadian and ultradian rhythms. By tuning into these natural highs and lows throughout the day, it is possible to use food to enhance or alleviate your mood.

As explained in the previous chapter, our mental and physical performance and energy levels follow a preplanned programme – but it is obvious that we don't all run to exactly the same biological clock.

Do you ever wonder why you don't feel at your best first thing in the morning, but can cope with late nights, whilst others have collapsed much earlier? There are some people who feel dreadful first thing in the morning, and yet can work well late into the night. This is because our internal clocks that regulate our circadian rhythms can vary from person to person by up to three hours – and is also the reason why some of us have to be forced out of bed! If you fit into this category, you are an 'owl', or an 'afternoon' person. Those who can leap out of bed immediately are described as 'larks' or 'morning' people. These people feel particularly groggy in the afternoon and find themselves reaching for sugary snacks! As you are now aware, this is the wrong thing to do. Even a healthy carbohydrate lunch will increase serotonin production in the brain and only add to the lethargic low you will be feeling anyway. If it is not practical to go and have a rest and you really need to keep going throughout the afternoon, then the answer is to eat protein foods at midday. This is power lunching. As carbohydrates calm you down, protein can help to energize the mind.

Following a protein meal or light snack, the brain is flooded with the amino acid tyrosine. This is used to make the brain chemicals dopamine and noradrenalin (norepinephrine). These neurotransmitters trigger brain cells that enhance concentration and mental alertness.

If you want to plan your meals to enhance brain chemistry when you need to keep alert and prevent a mental slump, choose the following high-protein foods:

- Any type of fish or shellfish
- Chicken or turkey meat – without the skin
- Low or medium fat cheese – such as cottage cheese, Edam, Gouda, Jarlsburg
- Very lean meat – ham, pork, lamb, bacon
- Soya-based products, such as tofu
- Plain yogurt, milk or soya milk
- Eggs.

If you are an afternoon person, but need to kick-start your day, choose a protein breakfast for a morning mental boost. If you are already highly charged and need to be calm, you can use carbohydrate foods to de-stress. A starchy breakfast and carbohydrate mini-meals throughout the day is a great way to maintain energy levels, keep calm and curb anxiety.

Use the principles of food and mood to suit your lifestyle and personality. Start by deciding if you are a morning or afternoon person. Check the basic menu plans to find out which type of foods are most suitable for you, and when. Remember, all foods contain a mixture of nutrients (except refined sugar and fats), but many foods will provide the majority of Calories from a single nutrient – either carbohydrate, protein, fat – or alcohol!

The basic meal plans described below are characterized by the major nutrients.

Morning Person Menu Plan

Drink a large glass of water (preferably bottled or filtered) before breakfast.

Meal	Major Nutrient
Breakfast	Carbohydrate
Morning snack	Carbohydrate
Power lunch	Protein
Afternoon snack	Protein
Evening meal	Carbohydrate
Snack – if required	Carbohydrate

Afternoon Person Menu Plan

Drink a large glass of water (preferably bottled or filtered) before breakfast.

Meal	Major Nutrient
Breakfast	Protein
Morning snack	Protein
Lunch	Carbohydrate
Afternoon snack	Carbohydrate
Evening meal	Carbohydrate
Snack – if required	Carbohydrate

Breakfast Foods

What to eat for a carbohydrate breakfast? There is plenty of choice here! Choose one or a combination of the following – depending on your energy needs.

- Wholemeal toast with scraping of butter or margarine, honey, jam or marmalade.
- Glass of fruit juice or tomato juice.
- Large bowl of porridge (choose organic jumbo oats soaked overnight with water). Serve with semi-skimmed milk and honey or brown sugar (for flavour and sweetness). If time is short, use instant porridge with hot milk. Choose original, or try fruit and nut variety. Avoid the chocolate-flavoured and heavily sweetened ones!
- High fibre/low sugar cereal such as Bran Flakes, Weetabix, Shredded Wheat, unsweetened muesli or even cornflakes. Add dried fruits or chopped banana for a change. Try muesli soaked overnight with fruit juice.

Protein Breakfast

- Grilled lean-back bacon and poached egg.
- Grilled kippers.
- Scrambled egg with grilled tomato, or smoked salmon.

Many people cannot face food first thing in the morning – or simply don't get up early enough to cook, prepare or eat breakfast. This is when they reach for a cup of coffee – with plenty of sugar – to get them going. As explained earlier, the brain needs a steady supply of glucose for peak mental performance, not a sudden dose of an artificial stimulant in the form of caffeine and a slug of sugar. Sudden changes in brain sugar levels lead to a hyperactive mind followed by depression. The answer, perhaps, would be to have nothing at all, but there is plenty of evidence to show that even a very small snack can boost your system, make you feel better and improve concentration.

So, if you normally reach for coffee to 'get you going' in the morning, try drinking a glass of water, a cup of tea (herb, fruit, green or weak black tea with lemon) and a glass of fruit juice and/or vegetable juice. Invest in a juicer and create your own fruit and vegetable juices, e.g. carrot and orange, carrot and apple. Prepare these the night before and enjoy them chilled the next morning. The fructose which fruit contains, as explained earlier, is absorbed more slowly and metabolized differently from ordinary sugar (sucrose), although both of these sugars are ultimately converted to glucose, which is metabolized to provide energy. This process is dependent upon the action of several important vitamins and minerals, in particular the B-vitamins and vitamin C. Fruit juice (especially blended with vegetable juices) will provide these, and the whole package will boost your mental performance and improve concentration in the morning.

Here are some other ideas to try:

- A handful of nuts – toasted almonds and hazelnuts, walnuts or peanuts.
- Whizz up a protein milk shake – milk with tinned or fresh raspberries or strawberries with a drizzle of honey if preferred.
- A pot of fruit yogurt or fromage frais.
- A glass of tomato juice.

Snacks

Carbohydrate	Protein
Toasted oatcakes and honey.	Toasted oatcakes and lean ham.
Fruit scone with scraping of butter, jam or honey if preferred.	Cheese scone.
Banana.	Melon or papaya with lime juice, and a small piece of cheese.
Ready to eat, moist apricots, figs, dates or prunes.	A handful of toasted almonds.
Wholemeal fruit muffin.	Fruit yogurt, or make your own by adding fruit purée and toasted sunflower seeds to natural yogurt.

Bowl of high fibre/ low sugar breakfast cereal.

Fresh fruit salad with fromage frais and toasted, flaked almonds.

Carbohydrate Lunches or Evening Meals

- Fresh spinach pasta with pesto or olive pastes.
- Baked potato with tuna fish or baked bean filling and green salad.
- Lentil, broth or vegetable soup with hunk of fresh crusty bread and scraping of butter or tahini (sesame seed paste).
- Macaroni cheese with leeks and onions.
- Fish pitta pockets – chopped mackerel, tuna or sardines mixed with natural yogurt and stuffed into pitta bread with chopped lettuce, watercress and tomato.

NB: If more fish filling is used in a small pitta bread pocket this could also be a protein meal.

Mental Power Eating – Protein Lunches or Evening Meals

- Chicken kebabs marinated in soya sauce and lime juice, served with steamed green vegetables.
- Cauliflower and broccoli cheesy bake.
- Avocado salad with walnuts and flaked, toasted almonds.
- Stir fry risotto with prawns, chicken, Quorn or tofu.
- Poached salmon or trout with steamed broccoli, and vegetable stir-fry.
- Bean bourgignon (bean and vegetables in a red wine casserole).

Energy Foods to Stock Up With/ Add to Your Shopping Trolley

We eat foods, not nutrients. The list below includes foods which will provide many of the energizing nutrients described earlier. They are foods which represent a good nutrient package, and adding them to your carbohydrate staples means that you are surrounded by foods which provide the basis of good eating patterns!

- Ready to eat (no need to soak) packets of apricots, figs, prunes and dates.
- Tins of fruit compote, pears, apricots, strawberries (canned in fruit juice rather than heavy – or light – syrup). Add to natural yogurt or whizz in a milk shake.
- Almonds, hazelnuts, walnuts, sunflower seeds – to add to salads, breakfast cereals, yogurts.
- Tinned beans to add to home-made soups, casseroles or vegetable and bean bakes.
- Fresh or frozen fruits and vegetables. Use chopped, frozen mixed vegetables as the basis for a quick home-made soup; sweetcorn, green and red peppers to throw into a quick stir-fry. Pick your own soft fruits in the summer and freeze a good stock of them.
- Green or black olives – a superb healthy nibble, if you like them.
- Try different breads – sesame and sunflower, walnut and sultana, date bread, rye bread, multigrain bread.

Sugar, Sunshine and Sadness

Optimum levels of serotonin can help to control appetite, and keep us happy, but the onset of winter, with its short dreary days brings with it depression, fatigue and weight gain for countless people who suffer from SAD (seasonal affective disorder). This is now a recognized disorder directly related to a lack of sunlight. This in turn is associated with a low level of serotonin, and here we have returned full circle to sadness because, as we know, when the level of serotonin drops too low, depression sets in. It is a morbid but relevant fact that there are more suicides in January than any other month of the year. Nevertheless, for the rest of the population who don't suffer from the full blown symptoms of SAD, winter is a time when we tend to feel definitely below par. There is nothing particularly wrong, you just lack sparkle and vitality. What is more, we find ourselves wanting to eat more – particularly carbohydrate foods, and not surprisingly we find that we have put on weight over the winter months.

The Bright Solution

The good news is that it can all be corrected – and the cure is free. Just as we need fresh air, good food and pure water for vitality, it is clear that another element should be added to the list – natural daylight.

What in the world does daylight have to do with appetite and mood? It seems that there is more to daylight than meets the eye, as extensive research carried out over the past 10 years in Europe and the USA has revealed. As well as enabling us to see, light also has its influence on our pineal gland. This is a tiny area at the base of the brain, about the size of a pea, which is very sensitive to light. It produces some very powerful chemicals which act as the central control for many physiological functions in the body. The melatonin which is secreted by this gland is a vital natural trigger for a number of other hormones which in turn regulate our growth patterns, cycles of metabolism, fertility, mood and appetite, and researchers have discovered that SAD sufferers endure a desynchronization of these body cycles during the winter months. The symptoms of depression and fatigue that they experience can be successfully treated using substitute daylight.

But what about the rest of us who, perhaps, do not suffer from SAD, but from November to February may be short of energy simply from the lack of daylight? In the depth of winter we go to work in the dark and come home in the dark. In between, we are cooped up under fluorescent lighting and, because of cold weather, we may not go outside so much. Even on a dull day the intensity of natural daylight is far greater than the artificial light we use in our homes and offices. Indoor lighting is on average a mere 500 lux, compared with light outside at 5000 lux. Also, indoor light does not have the same full spectrum of wavelengths, so is not the same as daylight to our brain.

With less light reaching the pineal gland, more melatonin is produced. Melatonin has been described as chemical sleep, so no wonder we feel drowsy and lethargic during the winter days. There is a link between light and the other soporific neurotransmitter, serotonin. Melatonin is produced from serotonin, so surges of the sleep chemical (from a lack of daylight) puts a drain on brain serotonin concentration. Low levels of serotonin make us feel depressed, moody and cause us to reach for a sugary fix in an effort to restore our serotonin levels.

How to Lighten Your Life

If you are fed up with being fed up during the winter months, and you are feeling the effects of those few pounds that you put on – even before Christmas – there is a solution which includes the basic meal plans outlined earlier.

- Most of your meals and snacks in a day should be based on the starchy, complex carbohydrate foods. This will maintain serotonin production.
- Eat protein meals only to improve alertness and concentration when you particularly need this (equivalent to power lunches for morning people, protein breakfast for afternoon people).
- Take a daily walk outside to put the natural light back in your life. Aim to spend a total of at least two hours outside each day. This could be made up of several half-hour walks. Even if it seems dull and grey outside, the full spectrum light you will be receiving will be significantly brighter than the artificial light you have left behind inside. A daily dose of natural light will help to curb the release of melatonin which would otherwise make you sleepy.
- If you cannot get outside, buy a lightbox which can sit on your desk for a few hours and provide the boost that you need. However, you would miss out on the benefits of exercise and the increased oxygen supplies enjoyed by a half-hour walk!

Some office workers have taken to using lightboxes, and they have been found to be particularly useful for shift workers. These people when they start a new shift, are having to do a good job and be productive at a time when their body and mind craves sleep. No wonder they are prone to fatigue, mild depression, irritability and lapses of concentration as their natural daylight cycles do a 12-hour flip and adjust to their new 'day'. A group of newsroom workers were asked to sit in front of a lightbox producing 10,000 lux for 30 minutes each evening before going to work. The effects were superb. Everyone found that the light therapy increased their alertness during their shift, and some even reported feeling more sociable and better tempered!

5
Fatty Issues

Fat is a concentrated source of Calories. (A Calorie is the unit for energy. It is a unit of heat which is used as a measurement of the amount of energy that has been released after foods are burnt (metabolized) in the body. The metric equivalent of this is the Joule and it is acceptable in most countries to use either of these units. Food labels give the amount of energy in the product as Joules (kJ) and Calories (kcal); 1 Calorie = 4.2 Joules.) One gram of fat provides 9 Calories compared with only 4 from carbohydrate (and 7 from alcohol). This is very useful when you need a food that will provide the maximum number of Calories with the minimum weight. A man doing hard physical work will burn about 3,600 Calories, but sitting all day at a desk requires only 1,800–2,500 Calories.

Everyone knows that a high-fat diet carries a risk of heart disease, and you are most at risk if you lead an inactive, sedentary life – so frequently the case in the business world. All the thinking, planning and concentration that is done in offices simply does not use up many Calories. It is physical work that counts. If, for instance, you were setting out to pull a sledge across the Antarctic, taking with you high-fat rations would be the only practical way to get enough Calories. But, if you are not, then too much fat will slow you down both mentally and physically. There can't be many people who have missed the message that the average Western diet is too high in fat and that a change is long overdue. The great news is that if you make the switch and change the types of foods that you are eating (from fatty foods to enjoying more carbohydrate foods) this one change has a triple benefit. Cut the fat and you'll be more alert, lose weight and have more energy. Let me explain each one in turn.

High-Fat Foods Slow the Brain

Recent research at Sheffield University's Human Nutrition Centre has shown that fatty foods slow down the brain and impair mental function. Scientists tested the performance of 18 volunteers after feeding them high-fat and low-fat midmorning breakfasts and lunches. The high-fat late breakfast was even worse than the high-fat lunch, leaving people tired, sluggish and easily muddled three hours later. It seems that when the digestive system is awash with a greasy mixture – alertness, accuracy and speed of completing tasks which require sustained attention is reduced. Even when people consumed more Calories in a high-carbohydrate, low-fat meal, their mental function was not as impaired as by a high-fat meal but with fewer Calories. A pork pie, slice of salami pizza or a cheese sandwich and packet of crisps may seem like an innocent snack, but if you want to stay sharp and mentally alert – stick to the carbohydrate or protein regimes described in Chapter 4.

Not All Calories Are Equal

If you make the switch, i.e. cut the fat and eat more carbohydrate foods, you are in severe danger of losing weight and having more energy! The reason behind both of these effects is because fat and carbohydrate are metabolized differently.

Energy is released from carbohydrate quickly to keep up with energy demand – which is especially important during exercise (see Chapter 6). Fat is metabolized much more slowly. The energy chugs out at a steady speed compared with the rapid pulse of energy from carbohydrate. Any excess fat that you may eat above your lack-lustre needs are also easily stored in adipose tissue and contribute to an expanding waistline! This is not the case when it comes to piling your plate high with carbohydrate foods. This is because, when it comes to putting on weight, not all Calories are equal. This needs some explanation.

The chemical name for the fat stored in your body is triglyceride. Most of the fat in the foods that we eat is also triglyceride. If we take in too much, it is a very simple process to deposit the excess on our thighs, hips and belly. A carbohydrate molecule, on the other hand, has a very different chemical structure from that of fat. Any excess carbohydrate must be broken down in the body and rearranged into a triglyceride. This process requires energy and is therefore an inefficient way of storing excess Calories because some are lost along the way. The equivalent of around 20 per cent of the original carbohydrate Calories are used up rearranging the molecule into fat which is then suitable for storage.

Fat Facts – The Inside Story

Fat has a very bad name, and rightly so – because we eat too much of it. Every year we swallow nearly three times our body weight in fat, and the consequences are clearly visible! It bulges from our bottoms or hangs in rolls from our waists and stomachs. It really does weigh us down in more ways than one. On the inside, what we don't see is the narrowing of blood vessels as fats get dumped in our arteries and clog the system. As everyone knows, this can result in a complete blockage of the artery, and if this occurs in one of the main arteries leading to the heart, it means a heart attack. If the smaller blood vessels in the brain are affected, the result is a stroke.

Not surprisingly, the cornerstone of healthy eating advice for the last 20 years, for populations across the affluent Western world, has been to reduce our total fat intake. This message is based on research which has defined a strong link between fat (particularly the saturated type) intake and diseases such as certain types of cancer, stroke and atherosclerosis. These can take many years to develop and a much more immediate effect of trying to function with a plumbing system with reduced bore pipes is that blood flow and therefore oxygen supply to every cell in your body is below its potential. No wonder we don't feel energized.

If asked, most of us would claim that we have cut down and that we don't eat much fat. The problem is that we tend to think of fats as blocks of butter and lard, or the stuff that drips from sausages and congeals in the grill pan after cooking. We prefer to overlook the huge hunks of cheese, dollops of mayonnaise, fried foods, pâté, burgers, real dairy ice-cream, biscuits, cakes or creamy sauces that we enjoy. All these are high-fat foods – but, more important, the type of fat they contain is saturated. This is important because when it comes to understanding fats, they probably cause more exasperation and confusion than any other aspect of nutrition.

There are no complications – the facts are simple; we are overdosing on saturated fats and yet are suffering from a deficiency of the unsaturated ones. These are strong words. In a modern affluent society no one would expect to be deficient in anything! First, let's deal with how saturated fats sabotage our circulation, and then the good news – how you can change things and even reverse the damage. It all centres around that substance called cholesterol.

The Truth About Cholesterol

When it comes to heart disease, cholesterol is the substance we fear most! This is understandable because when surgeons first cut open the arteries of those who had died of heart disease they saw yellow fatty deposits of cholesterol. The message seemed simple; avoid cholesterol and you won't get heart disease. And so, in an effort to be free of the fatty streaks that can harden and narrow our arteries in the process known as atherosclerosis, we go out of our way to avoid prawns, shrimps, egg yolks, liver and kidneys, which are the richest sources of cholesterol. It is only found in foods of animal origin, and yet some margarine manufacturers cash in on our paranoia and label their products 'low in cholesterol' even when they have been made from vegetable oils which would not contain it anyway!

The truth is that cholesterol is an absolutely essential substance in the body; it plays a crucial role in many areas of metabolism and is needed to form the membrane around every cell in your body. Because it is so essential, our liver manufactures all the cholesterol we need. In fact very little of the cholesterol that we eat is absorbed into the body. This means that cholesterol on our plate is relatively insignificant and makes very little impact on the concentration of cholesterol in the blood. Only a very small percentage of people in the population, those with an abnormal metabolism and very high cholesterol levels, need to worry about the amount of cholesterol that they eat. So, there is nothing wrong with cholesterol itself, the crucial part is in how it is metabolized. To blame cholesterol for clogging up our arteries and causing heart problems is rather like shooting the messenger. The real culprits are saturated fats, because they influence whether cholesterol finds its way into the artery walls – or not.

Cholesterol is a greasy, waxy substance that is transported around the body via the blood – which is mainly water. Everyone knows that oil and water don't mix, so cholesterol is attached to protein molecules. This cholesterol and protein particle is known as a lipoprotein and is the way that cholesterol is 'carried' in the blood. There are two main types of lipoprotein, Low Density Lipoprotein (LDL) and High Density Lipoprotein (HDL) that circulate in the bloodstream. The fate of the cholesterol they contain is very different. The LDL particles are harmful since they deposit excess cholesterol in the artery walls, causing them to narrow and harden. The HDL particles do the opposite, they are effectively 'Hoovers' sucking and removing cholesterol from the artery walls and taking it back to the liver out of harm's way. It is not difficult to realize that for the health of your arteries, it is a great advantage to have a higher proportion of HDL than LDL.

It used to be that your horoscope was a popular topic of conversation – nowadays it is your cholesterol number. A small finger-prick blood sample can be rapidly analysed in a simple cholesterol screening test, carried out routinely as part of lifestyle health checks. It is even possible to buy a DIY cholesterol-testing kit. Such has been the hype and the emphasis on knowing 'your number' that individuals may worry and become deeply stressed if it is above the desirable 5.5 mmol per litre (or 220 mg/dl). The truth is that a total blood cholesterol concentration is a very rough indicator of an individual's particular risk of developing heart disease. Other factors such as genetic susceptibility, smoking, high blood-pressure and lack of exercise also contribute to the overall risk. Moreover, if total cholesterol is high, the next step is to measure the lipoprotein fractions. If the concentrations of the harmful LDL particles is raised, this is an index of greater risk than a high HDL.

The good news is that it is possible to manipulate the levels of HDL and LDL floating around in your bloodstream. The most effective way of reducing the level of the 'bad' LDL is to eat less saturated fat in your diet. Platefuls of meat, cream, cheese, eggs, biscuits and ice cream is a sure way to push up your LDL particles! Another energizing change you can make to your lifestyle that will refresh your mind as well as clear the sludge from your arteries is regular exercise. This has the effect of increasing the concentration of the 'good' HDL particles.

A recent study carried out at the Stanford Centre for Research in Disease in California, added some new evidence to the exercise-cholesterol story and revealed that exercise can affect LDL levels as well. A group of 377 men and post-menopausal women, who had been diagnosed as having unhealthy cholesterol measurements, were divided into four groups and prescribed one of the following: a low-fat diet; an exercise regime; both a low-fat diet and exercise regime; no changes (this was the control group). Cholesterol levels were compared after a year. The individuals in the group who had followed the low-fat diet with exercise regime were found to have the biggest drop in the harmful LDL. Women who combined low-fat eating patterns with exercise cut their LDL cholesterol by an average of 14.5 mg/dl compared with a drop of 7.3 mg/dl for those who only reduced their fat intake.

It seems that exercise in tandem with a change in eating habits can not only increase the good HDL, but push down the bad LDL. The exercise regime used for the California study included at least 45 minutes of exercise (consisting of either jogging or fast walking) three times a week. A number of other studies have shown that exercise needs to be carried out regularly for at least four months before it will have a significant impact on cholesterol levels. It is common for regular runners and sportspeople to have quite a high blood cholesterol concentration, yet most of this is in the form of the protective HDL. The message is that a high total cholesterol does not mean that you are automatically heading for a heart attack; its all down to your lipoprotein fractions.

Another enjoyable way of increasing your HDL is a moderate alcohol intake – 'moderate' being the operative word! Around 4 units per day for men and 2 for women is the level that will have an effect. Any more than this and the effect is lost (added to which a high alcohol intake can contribute to obesity). It doesn't matter which alcoholic drink you choose, but as will be explained in the next chapter, red wine would be the best choice if you want a drink to help you unwind, or complement a good meal – as well as stacking up some health benefits.

Table 7. Calorie Content of Various Alcoholic Drinks

One unit of alcohol is equivalent to:

Drink	Calories
1 glass of dry red or white wine (12% alcohol)	75
1 glass of sweet white or sparkling wine (12% alcohol)	100

2 glasses of reduced alcohol wine (5% alcohol)	85
1 glass of rosé wine (12% alcohol)	80
1/2 pint of beer, lager or cider (4% alcohol)	100
1/4 pint of strong ale, cider or premium lager (6–7% alcohol)	95
1 measure of dry vermouth	55
1 measure of sweet vermouth	70
1 small glass of dry or medium sherry	55
1 small glass of sweet sherry	65
1 single measure of gin, whisky, brandy, rum, etc.	60

Essential Fats – A Cell's Golden Glow

In all this bad publicity one fact about fats gets ignored – some fats are vital, and we can't live without them.

We tend to think of fat merely as a concentrated source of Calories, but it is much more than that. Every nerve cell is coated in a layer of fat, and every cell in the body is defined by a fatty membrane. Chemically, all edible oils and fats are composed of units called triglycerides. These are made up of a glycerol 'backbone' onto which individual fatty acids are bonded. It is these fatty acids that are used to make cell membranes.

These are complex structures, and any engineer would be proud to have designed them. They are essentially two layers of fat with a layer of protein in between. The turnover of cells in the body is high; we are constantly making new cells to replace those which have died. Since fat is a vital ingredient for every cell, the types of fat that you eat will, sooner or later, show up in your membranes. Exactly what type of fats are available will determine the strength and vigour of each cell. This is because the fragile balance of fatty acids within the cell membrane determines whether it will resist, or encourage, disease. It is a bit like building a stone wall. If the pieces don't fit together well, the whole thing falls apart. Strong membranes constructed from unsaturated fatty acids can hold the cell together well and make it resistant to disease and the ageing process. If you normally eat a lot of butter, cheese, red meats, pâté, milk and cream, your cells will be flooded with saturated fat which will be used to make leaky membranes. If your cells are falling apart at the micro level, how can you expect to be fully functioning at the macro level?

Just think about it. If your cell structure, the very foundations of your organs – and ultimately your entire body – is constructed well, then this sends a golden glow and a strength throughout your whole being. Get the basic unit wrong and you are in all sorts of trouble. The latest theory about the cause of disease is based on how cells 'talk' to one another – and this communication depends on each cell having a strong membrane structure (i.e. constructed from unsaturated fats). Scientists have begun to unravel some astonishing facts about how it all works.

Cells – the Power Houses of Life

It's hard to think back that far, but all of us began life as a single cell. That cell then gets on with the business of dividing and replicating itself many millions of times into the adult being that others call 'you', and you call 'me'. Throughout the whole of our lives, as a child and then as an adult, there is constant built-in control over how our cells behave. Some cells must divide constantly so that hair and nails continue to grow and blood, skin and liver cells are laundered and replaced regularly. All this requires an intricate control system to regulate the destruction of some cells and the production of others. A team of scientists working at Aberdeen University have discovered how this is done. They believe that all cells are programmed to self destruct – unless they receive a signal from another cell to stay alive. By the time you have read this chapter, hundreds of millions of cells in your body will have died. You will survive this massive loss, though, because for every cell that dies, another will divide to replace it.

No one quite knows how the balance between cell death and cell division is achieved, but obviously it is vital if we are to avoid becoming totally overgrown or shrivel away to nothing. Clearly if each cell is programmed with a death wish and is also being kept alive by signals from other cells, communication between the cells is crucial! One essential aspect of this communication is via the cell membrane. This is not simply a barrier surrounding each cell, but a complex structure with the biological equivalent of farm gates, trap doors and letter boxes to allow certain substances in and out of the cell in a very controlled manner. Even within each cell are structures which in turn have their own membranes. The most important of these cell structures in terms of energy production are the mitochondria. These are known as the cell's power-houses, as this is where energy is finally released from the nutrients in the food we eat. Again, the membranes of these mitochondria are vital to their efficiency as energy producers. All this going on under our skin!

Fabulous Fats

These wonderful unsaturated fats that are so vital for every cell membrane are found in oily fish – such as mackerel, herring, pilchards, salmon, sardines, trout and tuna – olive oil, almonds and avocados. They are crucial for brain function –

60 per cent of the brain is made from fats, and most of these are unsaturated. The two fatty acids which are particularly potent are found almost exclusively in oily fish and have the tongue-twisting names of eicosapentaenoic acid (EPA) and docosahexaenoic acid (DHA). These are two of the omega–3 series of unsaturated fatty acids which are not only incorporated into the brain and other cell membranes, but are also needed to make very potent hormone-like substances called prostaglandins, thromboxanes and leukotrienes – collectively called eicosanoids. These have a number of beneficial effects. They can help to reduce high blood pressure and prevent migraines. They are powerful anticoagulants, helping to make the blood less 'sticky' so it flows freely within the arteries. Obviously, a blood clot, especially within the very fine, narrow blood vessels in the brain, would cause serious damage. The very low incidence of heart disease amongst the Japanese and traditional Eskimo populations may be explained by their high intake of oily fish and these omega–3 fatty acids.

Other eicosanoids work with the immune system and help to prevent inflammation reactions. This is particularly useful for anyone who suffers from irritable bowel syndrome (IBS), where stress and some foods can trigger the large bowel to become inflamed. Another type of inflammation causes the painful, swollen joints of rheumatoid arthritis. There have been many reports of sufferers seeing the painful swelling greatly reduced simply by including oily fish regularly in their diet.

There is another series of fatty acids, which are also important for health, known as the omega–6 series. These are not found in fish, but are concentrated in vegetable oils such as corn oil, safflower and sunflower oil, as well as in red meat from animals reared via the modern-day intensive production system (involving the use of concentrated feeds).

When all goes to plan, the omega–6 fatty acids act in balance with the omega–3s and together are just as essential to our bodies as vitamins. It is this balance which is vital, but unfortunately the foods we eat today have knocked the whole equilibrium out of kilter. When our bodies evolved they were nourished mainly by omega–3s with a smaller proportion of omega–6s roughly in a ratio of 4:1. Nowadays, with processed oils, margarines, dollops of mayonnaise, Big Macs and French fries the ratio has been flipped over and distorted dramatically – with disastrous results. Most of us are now eating far more omega–6s – the ratio is about 25:1. Cells overburdened with omega–6s convert them into arachidonic acid which in turn produces substances that are highly inflammatory, promote blood clotting and can trigger migraine headaches – the exact opposite to the benign effects of omega–3 which act to control metabolism and reduce cell damage.

The only way to correct the balance is to cut down dramatically on foods rich in omega–6 fatty acids and eat much more oily fish instead (white fish, such as cod or haddock, fried in batter, does not count!). Once fatty acids are eaten they are rapidly metabolized in the body, which means that a daily serving of oily fish will have a fairly immediate impact on tissues. Arthritis sufferers have noted an improvement (relief of soreness, stiffness and joint pain) after only 72 hours of eating oily fish each day.

Simple Steps to Increase Omega–3 Fatty Acids

- The deep sea cold water fatty fish (mackerel, herring, anchovies, salmon, sardines and tuna), are the richest sources of omega 3s (see Table 8). Lake trout, swordfish, turbot and shell fish – shrimp, prawns, crab, lobster – have smaller amounts.

- The UK's favourite oily fish is tinned tuna, but unfortunately the fabulously high omega–3 content is removed by the canning process. Mackerel is a better choice as most of this is smoked rather than canned. Aim to eat mackerel once a week and other oily fish three times a week.
- To get the most benefit from the omega–3s, poach or bake the fish. Frying or adding other fat (such as vegetable oils – safflower, sunflower, peanut, or corn – which are high in omega–6s) will reduce the omega–3 potency.
- Other foods which contain fabulous fats are olive oil, almonds and avocados. Use olive oil as often as possible (especially to make salad dressing), relish an avocado regularly and nibble on five almonds every day. Although these are high-fat foods, they provide the right type of fat and should become part of your eating patterns instead of the saturated fats which clog your arteries, inflame your membranes and trigger migraine headaches.

Table 8. The Omega–3 Fatty Acid Content of Seafood

Fish	Amount	Contents (mg)
Mackerel, smoked	2 small fillets	5,850
Kipper, baked	2 fillets	5,010
Herring, grilled	2 small fillets	1,820
Anchovies, canned in olive oil	2 fillets	1,600
Sardines, canned in oil, drained	1 small tin	1,860
Sardines, canned in brine, drained	1 small tin	1,620
Tuna, baked	small steak	1,500

Crab, boiled	1 portion	1,085
Pink salmon, poached	small cutlet	1,005
Rainbow trout, grilled	1 whole fish	800
Tuna, canned in oil	large portion	700
Sea bass, poached	1 serving	650
Squid	1 small portion	550
Lobster	1 small portion	350
Cod, poached	1 large fillet	215

Source: McCance and Widdowson, Royal Society of Chemistry Data Base, Fish and Fish products supplement 1993 and US Department of Agriculture.

You Can't Beat a Bit of Butter!

The debate over which is best for health – butter or margarine – has been raging for years. Faced with the choice of butter, margarine or the latest 'healthy' low-fat spreads, the conflicting advice from manufacturers can leave you cold with confusion. The margarine and low-fat spread producers condemn butter for its high saturated fat content (which it has), and include the impressively healthy sounding buzz words 'low fat', 'lite' and 'high in polyunsaturates' on their labels. They fail, however, to acknowledge that butter is a natural product, made simply by churning cream, whilst margarine is a totally synthetic, highly processed and artificial food. The two main ingredients are oil and water (the aim with low-fat spreads is to include as much water as possible). The oils used are generally the cheapest, industrially refined ones (palm, sunflower, rapeseed, safflower or fish oils). These are promoted as healthy because they contain a higher proportion of polyunsaturated fatty acids to saturated ones. All is reasonably well at this point in the ethics of a margarine manufacturer. However, to make their products, the oils must be chemically converted to a solid which can be glooped into a tub and, later, spread on our bread. This conversion is achieved by the process of hydrogenation and, by law, if oil in any food is hydrogenated the label must say so.

Ingredients are listed in descending order of quantity so you can check to see where hydrogenated oil appears and gauge the hydrogenated fat content. As an easy guide, softer margarines are less hydrogenated than hard block varieties. But why bother? What is so special about hydrogenated fats? The food manufacturers don't tell you that in the process of hydrogenation a new type of fat is created, known as a trans-fatty acid. These are, at best, nutritionally useless and, at worst, positively harmful to health. Although they are unsaturated fats, the molecule has been distorted from its natural shape in the hydrogenation process. The body cannot recognize this alien configuration and so treats a trans-fatty acid in the same way as a saturated fat. Hydrogenated fats, therefore, have the same potential as saturated ones to cause blood to clot and the harmful LDL cholesterol to rise!

Even products made from better quality oils, such as olive oil, are distorted by hydrogenation, and the magic of those special omega–3 fatty acids is lost. Hydrogenated fats are also used to make cakes, biscuits, mayonnaise, ready-made creamy sauces, crisps and fried snack products. Partially hydrogenated oils are used for frying in most fast-food restaurants because they do not go rancid as quickly as the 'pure' oils. All in all, we may be consuming a significant amount of the unhealthy 'saturated' fats in the form of the chemically modified trans-fatty acids. No wonder we reach for the low-fat spreads in an effort to decrease our fat intake. These do have a lower fat content (30–40 per cent fat) than butter or margarine (80 per cent fat), because they are made by whipping hydrogenated oils with water. To force oil and water to mix, emulsifiers, thickeners and stabilizers are added. Chemical preservatives extend the shelf life of the product, whilst artificial vitamins try to restore those lost in processing. At this point this synthetic product resembles a white, greasy, tasteless substance – so colourings, flavourings and sometimes salt are added. At the end of the day there is little to distinguish it from the plastic tub in which it is sold! When it comes to spreading something on our bread, remember that although butter is a source of saturated fat, it is a natural product and wins hands down on flavour. The message is enjoy it; savour the taste – just eat less of it.

Forget the Fake Fats

In between indulging in the so-called forbidden foods, many of us go on the diet treadmill, which, until recently, meant eating as a penance cardboard-like fat-free foods. A few years ago, like low-Calorie manna from heaven, came the fake fat revolution. These fake fats are substances (some are synthesized from sugars or proteins) that can provide the creamy mouth-feel of fats but without the Calories. Suddenly the supermarket shelves held no fears and there were no more forbidden foods. Chocolate, cream cakes, biscuits, gateaux, ice cream, custards and puddings now came without the fat. The theory is that these foods would replace the greasy, Calorie-laden alternatives and we could indulge in all this guilt-free goodness and keep the bathroom scales in check. The reality is that it hasn't worked out like this. The food industry has been expanding on the profits from the low-fat revolution – but unfortunately so have we. According to UK government statistics, 16 per cent of women and 13 per cent of men are now obese – double the incidence five years ago – whilst almost half the population is overweight.

In the last five years, the average UK dress size for women has increased from 14 to 16. The food industry has done an excellent job in brain-washing us to accept just one message; fat is bad. As a result we have ditched every other health or nutritional consideration in pursuit of the belief that anything 'low fat' makes us thin and that fake fats are somehow 'healthy' foods. The food industry feeds this belief by spending a fortune on the research and development of an ever increasing number of synthetic fats and fat substitutes with which to produce new foods and add to the ever expanding range of fat-free delights.

The latest and potentially most damaging of the fake fats is called Olestra. It is made from vegetable oil and sugar, but the molecules are too large and tightly packed to be absorbed by the body, so it passes straight through. Whilst other fake fats can't be heated beyond a certain point before breaking down, Olestra can be used in frying, making foods as greasy as you like but with the reassuring knowledge that fat will pass straight through your body. Olestra has recently been approved for use only in snack foods in America (although it may soon be permitted for a range of other fried foods and a cooking oil for home use). This approval occurred despite a blaze of controversy and opposition from health professionals, but is yet to be sanctioned by the UK Ministry of Agriculture Fisheries and Food. Why all the furore you may ask?

Olestra's unique selling point is that it passes straight through your body, but when eaten in large quantities it causes what is charmingly described as 'anal leakage'. Individuals who have been trying Olestra have complained that it leaks, leading to stained underwear and an oily toilet. Nevertheless, the US Food and Drug Administration has allowed its use provided that Olestra-containing foods carry the government health warning 'Olestra may cause abdominal cramping and loose stools'. What is more, it takes with it the valuable fat-soluble vitamins A, D, E and K as well as the carotenoids which play such a vital role in protecting the body against free radical damage (see Chapter 7).

So, here we have a synthetic substance which, because it is not absorbed itself, inhibits the absorption of other nutrients which are flushed out of the body and down the toilet. What a crazy situation! Olestra and other fake fats should not be seen as the miracle cure for the growing obesity problem. Synthetic foods are deeply unfulfilling because they send the wrong signals to the brain. The messages to our appetite centre get garbled and confused when a food we associate with fat doesn't contain any. We lose touch with real hunger because the signals, released after eating, no longer guide and direct us towards making the best food choices. We end up eating 'mentally' relying on low-fat labels to guide us through the food maze. Studies have shown that the 'lite' and fat-free foods are so dissatisfying that we end up eating something to compensate. (The same is true of foods manufactured using artificial sweeteners. Some people become addicted to them in an effort to satisfy their need for sweetness. The solution lies not in another can of diet drink or sugar-free yogurt, but to reach for real foods which are naturally sweet).

Many of the foods containing fake fats are highly processed, requiring a cocktail of emulsifiers, stabilizers, thickeners and flavourings to replicate the mouth-feel and taste of the lost fat – which is another reason not to eat them. It is time to opt for a quality diet and not displace real foods with poor imitations of the genuine article.

The best way to control fat intake is to make the naturally low-fat (but nutrient-rich) foods such as fruits and vegetables, cereals, breads, pasta and rice the cornerstone of your eating habits. Then add in and enjoy smaller amounts of foods which are high in fat but provide as many of those omega–3 fatty acids as possible. Finally, if you enjoy foods with saturated fats, there is no need to eliminate them from your diet – or worse, feel guilty when you do eat them. Simply choose the best. Why settle for a chemically sweetened, reduced fat chocolate bar which tastes so artificial when you can relish real, top quality Belgian or Swiss chocolate? Chewing on rubberized, half-fat cheese is an insult to your taste buds compared with enjoying a really excellent, but small, piece of your favourite – and the finest – Cheddar, Stilton, Brie or Parmesan. We should be taking care over our food, like the Italians and French, cooking it with love, appreciating its quality and eating it for its flavour!

Annotated Executive Menu

Starters

Pâté: Chicken livers are low in fat but pâté contains a high proportion – which is saturated fat. Duck pâté is very rich as duck meat is extremely fatty. Choose smoked mackerel pâté, which has proportionally more of the omega-3 fatty acids than meat or poultry based ones.

Oatcakes: good choice. They go well with the pâté and provide some useful dietary fibre.

Chicken Liver Pâté
and Toasted Oatcakes

Avocado Vinaigrette

Prawn Cocktail

Hummus

Taramasalata

Soup of the Day

Avocado: Wonderful choice! Bursting with unsaturated fat and vitamin E. Enjoy, relish and feel the goodness soothing each cell and revitalizing your body.

Prawn Cocktail: The prawns are a good source of omega-3 fatty acids, but the mayonnaise is very rich in omega-6s. Ask for a cocktail with the mayonnaise separately which you can use as a dip rather than poured over the prawns. You'll end up eating about a third less of the mayonnaise.

Hummus: Famous Middle Eastern chickpea pâté with garlic, lemon juice and tahini (sesameseed paste) and olive oil. The tahini and olive oil provide the high fat content (310 Cals from fat per 100 g), but these are omega-3s and other unsaturated fats.

Soup of the Day: Avoid 'cream of' soups as these provide a lot of saturated fats. Choose vegetable based soups (for the vitamins) or broths with lentils, barley or split peas (for fibre and flavour).

Taramasalata: Made with cod's roe and olive oil which provide a lot of fat (510 Cals from fat per 100g) but, like hummus, the type is fat is unsaturated. To reduce your total fat intake, choose Tsatsiki instead (made from cucumber, onion, garlic and olive oil), which has similar flavours but a much lower fat content (40 Cals from fat per 100g).

Main Courses

Sea Food Risotto: A fabulously tasty and energizing dish. A wonderful mixture of low-fat fish with plenty of carbohydrate from rice.

Beef Casserole: Beware of the word 'rich' as the meat is likely to contain a higher fat content than lean meat used for steaks. Ostrich, venison and rabbit meat have a lower fat content.

Sea Food Risotto

A delicate mixture of prawns, shrimps, squid, mussels with diced vegetables and wild rice

Beef Casserole

A rich casserole of local beef with vegetables in a red wine gravy

Grilled Rainbow Trout: The perfect way of cooking any fatty fish which are oozing with those wonderful omega-3 fatty acids. The flaked almonds also have unsaturated fat.

Grilled Rainbow Trout

Fresh trout with flaked almonds

Chicken Kiev: Chicken and Turkey are low-fat meats as most of the fat is concentrated in a layer under the skin. Removing the skin before cooking (except roast meats), means 12 per cent less fat and 30 per cent fewer Calories. Beware, with Kiev the fat content is greatly increased by adding garlic butter and frying.

Chicken Kiev

Supreme of chicken stuffed with garlic butter, coated in breadcrumbs and deep fried

Cold Poached Salmon

Best available salmon served with dill mayonnaise and cucumber

Cold Poached Salmon: Those wonderful omega-3s again, but beware of the mayonnaise which will cancel out their benefit by providing a dollop of omega-6s.

Vegetable stir fry: Another perfect choice. Stir-frying hardly uses any fat at all. Relish the flavours and colours of the vegetables – which because they are cooked so quickly are also bursting with vitamins.

Spicy Vegetable Stir Fry

Fresh vegetables stir-fried with selected spices and served on a bed of rice

Broccoli Quiche: A classic dish for vegetarians, but beware, the cheese and pastry contribute a lot of saturated fat to this healthy sounding creation.

Broccoli Quiche

Cheese, onion, Broccoli and egg flan

Vegetable Stroganoff

A selection of vegetables simmered in cream, paprika and brandy

Vegetable Stroganoff: Beware the double cream, it provides a lot of saturated fat in an otherwise vibrant mixture of ingredients.

Mushroom and Nut Piquant

Mushrooms sautéd in a garlic butter with ginger, onions, peanuts, sesame seeds and soya sauce and served on a bed of noodles

Mushroom and Nut Piquant: Provided that not too much butter is used to sauté the mushrooms, the remaining ingredients – especially garlic, onions and ginger – contain fabulously energizing compounds (see Chapter 7).

Side Dishes

Roast potatoes soak up a lot of saturated fat if cooked in the same pan as the meat joint. A crunchy crispy healthy alternative is to brush par-boiled potatoes with olive oil and 'roast' in a separate pan at a high oven temperature. Choose thick cut, straight French fries – they have a lower surface area compared with thin or crinkle-cut potato strips, which means they absorb less fat when fried.

Vegetables – carrots, spinach, etc. Ask for them to be un-glazed as most are served with melted butter.

Roast potatoes or French fries

Carrots, spring greens, spinach

Roll and butter

Green salad with French dressing

Roll and butter: A wholemeal roll will provide 5 grams of fibre, a white one only 2 grams. Enjoy the flavour of butter, but to make a little go a long way, use it at room temperature. It will spread thinly and you'll use at least 50 per cent less.

Green salad: Eat as much of this as you can! Ask for the French dressing to be served separately so that you can regulate the amount used, or try a squeeze of lemon and black pepper.

Desserts

Death by Chocolate:
Full of saturated fat and sugar – but if you have saved your saturated fat 'points' until now, make sure that you enjoy it to the full. And remember, you don't have to finish the whole serving – which is usually enough for two!

Crême Caramel:
Made with milk and eggs – two ingredients which provide saturated fat – but a small portion is wonderful!

Death by Chocolate
Layers of chocolate sponge with ice-cream and chocolate sauce topped with, toasted nuts and flakes of Belgian chocolate

Crême Caramel

Fresh Strawberries and Cream

Melon:
Any fresh fruit is a wonderful low-fat choice – especially if you have already enjoyed the higher fat dishes.

Melon with Raspberry Coulis
Fresh melon strips served on a bed of raspberry purée

Selection of Cheese and Biscuits

Strawberries and Cream: Clotted cream has the highest fat content (52 per cent), followed by double cream (48 per cent), whipping cream (38 per cent), single cream (22 per cent). Switching to Greek yogurt (12 per cent), natural yogurt (3 per cent) or Fromage Frais (3 per cent) will have a significant effect on your fat intake – but not the enjoyment.

Cheese and Biscuits:
Go easy with the cheese as their total fat content is of the highly saturated type. Cheddar (35 per cent fat), soft cream cheese (47 per cent), Danish Blue (30 per cent), Stilton (36 per cent), Feta (20 per cent), Edam (22 per cent), Jarlsberg (23 per cent). Watch out for the biscuits too – oatcakes or waterbiscuits are the best choice.

6

Gain the Edge through Exercise

Not being active is a real waste of our human potential. To the ancient Greeks, exercise was a vital part of daily life. The historian Xenophon said that it is a 'disgrace for a man to grow old without seeing the beauty and the strength of which his body is capable'. Unfortunately, the attitude of today's workforce is very different. Only 20 per cent of all office workers take regular exercise and yet those who do are the ones with the most energy!

If we know that regular exercise is good for us, why do we do so little of it? Could it be that we are doing it for the wrong reasons? Those who are motivated to take exercise through guilt or because their doctor, partner, children, friends or colleagues told them they should, will have a hard time of it. Exercise then becomes a penance, something to be endured and 'got over with' as quickly as possible. This is not good, since the essence of exercise is to integrate the mind with the body. Wherever your mind goes, your body and behaviour follows. The trick is to take your mind with you when you exercise your body, so that whatever the activity it becomes a total (and enjoyable) mind-body experience. In his book *Body, Mind and Sport*, John Douillard explains that:

> *In our society we pride ourselves on how many things we can do at one time or accomplish in one day. In ancient times,*

pride was taken in the quality of the accomplishment rather than for the accomplishment itself. There is an old saying: A painter paints with his hand, an artist paints with his hand and his mind, and a master paints with his hand, his mind and his heart. It is the same with all things. If our entire focus isn't on what we are doing, no matter how simple the job, the result will be compromised.

The exercise that will do you most good is one which you enjoy doing – not the one you endure. So, if you want to do aerobics or circuit training or whatever, find a class that is fun! Choose an instructor who makes every session into a party! Make exercise a social event – pile into the bar afterwards for an après-sweat fruit juice, and chat about how great you feel! It seems taboo to talk about actually enjoying exercise – the conversations tend to revolve around your latest strained muscle, pulled tendon or blister. If this is your attitude, change it – or try something new. The latest popular craze of line dancing involves a lot of moving about to music, and is great exercise, but look at the faces of experts and beginners alike – it is clear that they are having fun!

Be warned, the toughest part about taking regular exercise is getting started. Ask anyone, from superfit athletes to regular runners (who thoroughly enjoy being active), and they'll all say the same; the hardest part about taking exercise is getting changed and past the front door! It's that half-an-hour before you've planned to go out to run/swim/cycle, and the smallest excuse is likely to stop you. Breaking out of this comfort zone may be a challenge, but it is worth it. The hectic life of business demands a mind that is sharp, with good mental skills and powers of concentration. Exercise gives you the edge because being physically fit means being mentally fit.

International athlete, Ron Clarke in his book *Total Living* explains that...

> *...if your body and soul are properly toned, you can cope with a greater variety of 'the good life' than normal. The feel of a taut, tight body able to undertake any task with ease, a mind that can concentrate for six to ten hours at a time, a spirit which is always up, a temperament which copes equally well with the triumphs and disasters of daily business, not to mention family life, are all products of a simple, daily concern for not-very-long workouts and nutritional value in your meals.*

Executives, Entrepreneurs and Exercise

Britain's business leaders are generally not a healthy lot. Their most feverish activity is the endless networking over lunch and playing an occasional game of golf. However, a growing number of top businessmen are joining many thousands of more ordinary folk in the challenge of marathon running. One of the best known 26-milers in the business world is Sir Rocco Forte, until recently Chairman of the Forte hotel and restaurant group. He has completed eight marathons – seven in London and one in New York. Most runners aim to run up to 60 miles a week for three months before the big day. This eats into around 10 hours every week, which represents quite a commitment for any busy person. When that person is the head of a multinational company, working up to 70 hours each week, it takes an impressive dose of time management to fit in the training. Forte obviously makes it a priority and an essential part of his business life. 'I like being fit. If I'm not fit I am not on form and don't have as much stamina.' Other business marathon executives claim that they have some of their best business ideas while out running. When you are pounding round the local park, there are no phones ringing, faxes dropping on your desk or meetings to disturb your thinking.

Except for the elite runners who compete to win, 10-kilometre runs, half-marathon or full-marathon events are non-competitive. It is an internal challenge that you are facing. Getting yourself fit enough to complete an organized event, unlike climbing Everest, is not terribly difficult. Desperately hard work, yes; difficult, no. It is like giving up smoking, perfectly possible if you really want to do it; impossible if you don't. The marathon or any of its shorter versions have become the great attainable goal of suburban life. To enjoy the challenge and compete against yourself brings lasting benefits along the way as well as on THE day.

No Pain, No Gain?

Although exercise greatly reduces stress, it is surprising how many conventional sports practices actually contribute to it. The popular phrase 'no pain, no gain' only encourages the view that exercise means suffering. Pain is the body's way of communicating that something is wrong, and yet we are told to ignore it and simply run through it – until the body is positively screaming at us to stop. By this time the damage is done and there is usually a knock-on effect in other parts of the body. This is when exercise adds to, rather than dissolves, stress. The alternative is to listen to your body during exercise and to stay within the comfort zone. This means that when a pain comes, slow down your pace until you feel comfortable. Ironically it is the body's response to severe pain that can give us a false sense of security and add an incredible amount of stress through our exercise habits.

Runner's High

It starts harmlessly enough, we want to push ourselves that little bit further each time, but once we stop listening to bodies the benefits of the mind and body connection are lost. Many serious runners become obsessed with the finish line in a long race, or simply want to exercise each day. Onlookers can only wonder at what drives them on at such a pace, especially whilst suffering from heat exhaustion, sore shins, painful knees or raw blisters. The answer is that it is a strange sense of euphoria, otherwise known as 'runner's high', that gets them to the finish line. When the body is exhausted or in pain, it produces its own pain-killers to help the person endure the ordeal. These endorphins, enkeph-alons and other morphine-like substances act on the brain and are the same chemicals which are released when you experience pleasure. Endorphins have pretty much the same effect as injecting yourself with morphine – except that this free shot of bliss comes from within. The dramatic absence of pain is enthralling, but it means that your body is dissociated from your mind. You feel inspired, have momen-tum, you are unstoppable. It is as though you have slipped into cruise control – moving along is almost effortless, it seems like flying. You are, in short, addicted to your own endorphins. This can be self-defeating for some individuals if the level of exercise that they need to do to produce this effect is greater than their body can cope with.

How Much Exercise?

The common feature for any goal in life is that there is always a path to it. Sometimes it is a long one, and it is impor-tant to realize this. This helps you resist the temptation to look for quick-fix solutions to a weight problem or fitness. When it comes to exercise (or changing your eating habits), it is important to make the journey along the path so appealing that it becomes as enjoyable as the achievement itself. This can be done by being aware of the progress that you are making, rather than only seeing your final goal.

Forget the notion that if a little exercise is good – a lot must be better. Like your eating habits, exercise is an individual matter. A certain pattern for one person might help to reduce their stress, but in another will only add to it. Nevertheless, some individuals will push their bodies beyond their own limits – and pay the price. Many dedicated runners suffer from more colds and infections than those whose schedule is less intense. Studies have shown that the optimum level of exercise for you as an individual gives the immune system a slight boost, but above this level and immune function is suppressed. This is because exercise produces a chemical called glutamine, which is the preferred fuel for white blood cells (which help engulf bacteria) and stimulate the immune system. After extreme exertion, such as running a marathon or over-training (for example, by running 50 miles per week when your body is only ready to handle 25 miles) glutamine levels plummet, ultimately leaving you more prone to infection.

A way to check that you are working at the right intensity for you is to monitor your pulse. There are plenty of heart-rate monitors on the market which will give you a continuous reading of your on-going heart rate on a device that looks like a wrist watch. A cheaper alternative is to take your pulse manually either at the wrist, the temple or carotid artery on the neck. Exactly which intensity is the best one to work at for general fitness has been the subject of controversy for several years. The advice used to be that 70 per cent of your own maximum heart rate was the intensity that brought maximum results. This was based on the old 'no pain, no gain' school of thought, and several studies carried out at the University of North Carolina's Cooper Institute for Aerobic Research have shown that young healthy male subjects who exercised at 50 per cent of their predicted maximum showed significant improvement in their aerobic fitness. The men exercised for 30–40 minutes, 5 days a week for 10 weeks.

Most magazine articles on the benefits of exercise will advise you to work at around 65–85 per cent of your maximum. This is because we expect to push ourselves when we exercise and we want fast results. But if you want to enjoy taking exercise and revel in the gain and not the pain, the 50–60 per cent zone will bring the same benefits that higher exercise intensities will bring. The frequency of exercise is also important, a brisk two-mile walk with your dog every day is much better than thrashing around a squash court at 80 per cent of your maximum once every three weeks.

Use the following formula to work out 50–60 per cent of your maximum heart rate to find your training zone.

> The first thing to do is to measure your resting pulse, and the best time to take this is first thing in the morning. With the palm of your hand upwards, gently press two fingers at the base of your thumb where your wrist bone is. Usually the palm line that curves around the thumb area ends just above the spot where you can feel your pulse. Count the pulse for 15 seconds (taking the first beat as zero) and then multiply by four to get your resting pulse rate.
>
> Your optimal training heart rate is then 220, minus your age, plus your resting heart rate, times 50 per cent.

For example, the optimal training heart rate for a 32-year-old person with a resting heart rate of 66 beats per minute would be: 220 – 32 = 188 + 66 = 254 × 50/100 = 127 beats per minute.

To calculate 60 per cent of maximum for the same individual: 220 – 32 = 188 + 66 = 254 × 60/100 = 152 beats per minute.

Divide the final answer by 6 to give the number of beats per 10 seconds (which is easier to measure during exercise).

The aim for this person is to exercise at between 127 and 152 beats per minute or 21 to 25 beats every 10 seconds.

Resting heart rate is a good indicator of how fit you are. As you become fitter through regular exercise, your resting heart rate will decline. Use Table 9 to find out how fit you are and to chart your progress.

Table 9. How Fit Are You – Based on Your Resting Heart Rate?

Age	8–25		26–35		36–45		46–55		56–65	
Sex	M	F	M	F	M	F	M	F	M	F
Excellent	49–55	54–60	49–54	54–59	50–56	54–59	50–57	54–60	51–56	54–59
Good	57–61	61–65	57–61	60–64	60–62	62–64	59–63	61–65	59–61	61–64
Above Average	63–65	66–69	62–65	66–68	64–66	66–69	64–67	66–69	64–67	67–69
Average	67–69	70–73	66–70	69–71	68–70	70–72	68–71	70–73	68–71	71–73
Below Average	71–73	74–78	72–74	72–76	73–76	74–78	73–76	74–77	72–75	75–77
Poor	76–81	80–84	77–81	78–82	77–82	79–82	79–83	78–84	76–81	79–81
Very Poor	84–95	86–100	84–94	84–94	86–96	84–92	85–97	85–96	84–94	85–96

What Happens When You Exercise? The Inside Story

'Use it or lose it' is an old adage – but which bits do you use? Different activities contribute differently to health, but there are basically two types of exercise: anaerobic and aerobic. The latter is any sustained activity which forces your body to take up a great deal of oxygen. Running, swimming, rowing, cycling, dancing all improve cardiovascular fitness. That is they strengthen the heart, improve oxygen circulation and boost respiration. This is because aerobic exercise means endurance, and the only way you can keep going is to train your heart, lungs and circulation system to improve the delivery of oxygen to your muscles. Anaerobic exercises (weight lifting, circuit and resistance training) are the opposite, they do not involve prolonged, intensive breathing. They are stop and start activities and are good for building strength and flexibility, but the oxygen factor is not there. Their benefit is that they develop muscle tone and strength. A strong muscle is able to endure physical stress for longer. For example, simple weight training can strengthen back muscles and improve the mechanics of the vertebral column, helping to prevent back pain, slipped disc and sciatica.

In general, anaerobic exercise will improve the amount of force, or strength that your muscles can produce. This is useful for sports such as tennis, rowing, martial arts or boxing. Aerobic exercise develops your stamina and reflects your ability to keep going (see Table 10).

Table 10. Benefits from Exercise

Most activities will have an effect on your strength, skill, suppleness and stamina. This table highlights the main benefit for each activity.

Stamina
Aerobics
Swimming
Cycling
Walking
Step aerobics
Stair climber
In-line skating (roller blading)
Rowing
Kick boxing
Orienteering
(Circuit training)
(Squash)
(Skiing)
(Tennis)
(Dance)

Skill
Ice Skating
Skiing
Badminton
Netball
Hockey
Football
Martial Arts
Basketball

Strength
Weight Training
Circuit Training
Resistance training
with rubber tubing
(Step aerobics)
(Martial Arts)
(Rowing)
(Skiing)
(Swimming)
(Dance)

Suppleness
Yoga
Stretching exercises
(Martial Arts)
(Swimming)
(Kick Boxing)

The benefits of aerobic exercise extend far beyond the muscle strength.

Circulation, Heart and Blood Pressure

The reason why your resting heart rate decreases as you get fitter is because after a few months of regular exercise, the walls of your heart thicken and the force of each beat increases. The heart normally contracts 100,000 times each day, pumping 18,000 litres (3,960 gallons) of blood around the body. Clearly if more blood is pumped out for every heartbeat, the efficiency of the pump is increased and your resting heart rate can decline by up to 20 per cent. Regular exercise improves the ratio of the beneficial HDL cholesterol compared with the harmful LDL type. Studies have shown that if you run for about 145 minutes per week, you are around 40 per cent less likely, compared with a sedentary person, to have a heart attack. If you were overweight before you began to take exercise, it will help to trim your weight which in turn will lower your blood pressure and take some of the strain off your heart. If your weight was normal to start with, exercise will have a negligible effect on your blood pressure.

Muscles

In the beginning there is muscle soreness – the result of using muscles that you haven't used for a while. This can follow your first work-out or a day spent digging the garden. There are two types of muscle soreness: acute and DOMS (delayed onset muscle soreness). The former occurs during exercise and fades immediately afterwards.

The vigorous and forceful contractions of weight training or any resistance exercise reduces the blood flow to the muscle fibres which then hampers the muscle's ability to 'wash out' the by-products of metabolism. These include lactic acid and potassium which accumulate and stimulate the nerve endings – causing swelling and pain. DOMS, on the other hand, doesn't tend to hit you with full force until 24 hours after the exercise, and then the stiffness and pain can last for several days.

Despite plenty of research to investigate the changes that occur inside the muscle before, during and after exercise, no one has discovered the exact cause of DOMS – or come up with an effective cure! Obviously, some sort of damage to the muscle fibres has occurred, but this does not explain the 24-hour pain delay. It is puzzling that surgical operations, that involve cutting abdominal muscle, probably cause the same sort of damage – yet the pain is felt immediately. If you enthusiastically overdo the number of sit ups, your stomach muscles are certainly damaged – but the soreness is delayed.

When beginning an exercise programme, common sense can help prevent muscle soreness. Start gently and within your own comfort range. Make sure you have warm muscles before you start any vigorous exercise. The warm up and cool down phases should include a number of stretching exercises (which also improve flexibility). Concentrate on gently stretching the muscles, using a full range of movement, not bouncing which can cause muscle fibres to tear. DOMS is a self-limiting disorder and the soreness can be temporarily relieved by gentle stretching followed by a hot bath and/or a soothing massage which, it has to be said, are wonderful ways of recovering. Rest is probably the best approach. The golden rule, as discussed earlier, is to exercise at around 50 per cent of your maximum heart rate, listen to your body and do not attempt to work through the pain.

Tendons

Pound for pound the tendons (the fibres which join muscles to bone) have to endure considerable stresses during weight-bearing exercises. When you are relaxed there is 25 lb of pressure on the tendons around your lower back and knees. This rises to 100 lb when you are standing and 1,000 lb when running. Every time your foot strikes the ground you are putting three to four times your body weight on them. For a 10 stone person, that's up to 40 stones with every step! All runners should invest in a good pair of shoes which are designed to absorb some of the shock that would otherwise be transferred to their knees, hips and spine.

Skin

Exercise improves the circulation to the skin and your ability to sweat. Sweating is not related to fitness; some very fit people positively drip as soon as they start moving, whilst others eventually break sweat. Regular exercise improves our tolerance to heat and cold. It can help clear teenage skin conditions such as acne, eczema and psoriasis.

Enter the Fat-Burning Zone

Some people dedicate their lives to reducing their body fat content but a certain amount is required as a vital constituent of the nerves, spine, brain and cell membranes. Adult men have 3–5 per cent of this 'essential fat' and women have 10–12 per cent. The remaining fat content of the body is stored in adipose tissue and represents the main energy reserve – and the amount of excess Calories stored here can vary enormously between individuals. Whilst the desirable range of body fat content for a fairly sedentary 35-year-old man is 12–16 per cent, the average man is around 18 per cent – which is equivalent to 60 half-pound packs of butter! Similarly, the desirable range for a woman is 19–23 per cent, but statistics reveal the average is 26 per cent body fat.

Regular aerobic exercise can not only help to reduce body fat content, but can increase the proportion of lean muscle tissue as well. The significance of this change in body composition for weight control is that overall metabolic rate is increased. Muscle is metabolically active – compared with fat, it requires more Calories just to keep it ticking over. Most women worry about doing too much exercise for fear of building up too much muscle. An increase in muscle size is difficult for women because, compared to men, they have lower levels of the hormone testosterone. Women who do regular exercise will increase their muscle strength rather than size.

For complete beginners, just running for 30 minutes three times a week at a modest pace (eight or nine minutes per mile) will burn at least 1300 extra Calories per week. Provided that food intake does not increase, this can mean a loss of 17 lb of body fat in one year. During exercise, both fat and carbohydrate are burnt as fuels to provide energy. Proportionally more fat is burned at lower exercise intensities, and it was thought that half an hour's activity at this level would be more effective in shifting excess fat than busting a gut for 30 minutes at a more strenuous level.

This does not work in practice because weight loss depends on total Calories burned. Half-an-hour of strolling along a beach would burn around 150 Calories, whereas the same time spent briskly walking up a gentle hill would use up approximately 270. What is most relevant, however, is the duration and intensity of the exercise. A whole day walking in the hills will burn more Calories than a 40 minute jog. It is often easier to pack in more sessions of low intensity exercise than one thrashing, exhausting blast out! Beginners, especially, should aim to start, for example, on an exercise bike at a comfortable level for longer rather than going 'flat out' for a shorter time. Check the figures in Table 11 to see how sport and everyday activities compare.

Table 11. Calorie Cost of Sport and Everyday Activities

Activity	**Calorie cost per hour**	**Calorie cost per 10 minutes**
Aerobics	480	80
Aqua aerobics	480	80
Basketball	400	67
Cleaning the house	270	45
Climbing stairs	680	115
Circuit training	540	90
Cycling (relaxed)	300	50
Cycling (12 mph undulating)	660	110
Dancing (relaxed)	370	62
Digging the garden	500	83
Football	540	90
Judo or Karate	780	130
Jogging (10 mph)	360	60
Running (7 mph)	850	142
Rowing (competition)	900	150
Scrubbing the floor	410	68
Skiing, downhill	580	97
Squash	600	100
Swimming (front crawl)	510	85

Swimming (relaxed)	360	60
Tennis (recreational singles)	450	75
Walking (relaxed, 2 mph)	240	40
Walking (brisk, 4 mph)	360	60
Weeding the garden	210	35

These figures are estimations based on an individual weighing 68 kg (150 lb). For every 7 kg (15 lb) above this add 10 per cent to the Calorie figure, and subtract 10 per cent for every 7 kg below the 68 kg. To carry out the same activity, men will burn slightly fewer Calories than men of the same weight and age. The exact figure for an individual will depend on the precise intensity, style and technique used to carry out the activity.

Taking exercise is no longer something that you must confine to doing in your spare time. Workplace fitness and lifestyle programmes are increasingly popular in Britain and North America. Companies who provide sports facilities or have corporate gym memberships agree that the initial start up costs of such ventures have been far outweighed by the benefits – such as a decrease in employee turnover, reduced absenteeism and medical costs, and greater productivity. It is, therefore, much easier to integrate a lunchtime fitness class into your business routine and, of course, you can always walk or cycle to work!

Fuelling Your Muscles – What to Eat for Exercise

With the vast array of sports drinks and energy bars currently on the market you could be forgiven for assuming that an active person needs to consume these for fuel. Although they do have their uses, the best eating plan to fuel active muscles is based on those power-packed starchy carbohydrate foods (bread, pasta, rice, beans, lentils, root vegetables – especially potatoes – and porridge). These should be the foundation of most meals, so that you are fuelling your body with the right type of energy for active muscles. Then, if you need to fill an energy gap, a carbohydrate snack, eaten roughly an hour before exercise, will provide the final top-up. Exactly when you have this is down to personal choice, as some people can tolerate eating closer to exercise than others. The snack is particularly useful if you haven't eaten for several hours. It can even be a mini meal in itself depending on the demands of the exercise.

Suitable pre-exercise snacks include:

- A large banana, orange, pear or apple
- A handful of raisins or sultanas
- A small fruit scone with a little jam or honey
- A currant bun
- Two round oatcakes
- A fruit muffin
- A wholemeal bread roll filled with half a banana and a little honey
- A fruit or cereal muesli bar
- Six dried apricots
- A small pot of fruit yogurt.

Why Is Carbohydrate So Important for Exercise?

We have huge potential energy already stored in the body – as fat. Even a thin, lean, 70 kg (155 lb) man has around 75,000 Calories stored as fat – enough to keep him walking the equivalent of 23 marathons! Ms Average who is not overweight has around 102,000 Calories as fat. In contrast, we have a limited amount of carbohydrate – stored in the muscles and liver as glycogen. Ms Average has only 1,200 Calories and Mr Average only 1,600 Calories stored as glycogen – enough to fuel a couple of hours of squash. Unfortunately, the energy for most types of exercise is generated by burning mainly glycogen (which can be converted to glucose) rather than fat. This is because the energy produced from fat is released relatively slowly, which is fine for low intensity activities such as strolling along the beach or reading this book. As soon as we do anything more energetic we need a faster rate of energy production, and this comes from burning carbohydrate (glycogen and glucose).

Think of carbohydrate as the jet fuel for the body, it can be ignited to give an immediate and rapid supply of energy to keep up with demand. Fat is at the other end of the spectrum, as the peat burner, offering a prolonged, steady but more gentle source of energy. When your carbohydrate store runs out, fatigue sets in. This is when you feel tired, your legs and arms are heavy and it's a real struggle to keep going. To maintain power and drive throughout exercise you need to eat carbohydrate foods regularly beforehand so that you start with a full tank of jet fuel.

How Much Carbohydrate Do I Need?

The more active you are, the more of your Calories should come from eating carbohydrate. If you have just started taking exercise, you need 4.5 g of carbohydrate per kilogram of your body weight per day.

- For a 62 kg (137 lb) female, her minimum needs will be: $62 \times 4.5 = 279$ grams of carbohydrate per day.
- For a 70 kg (154 lb) man, his minimum needs will be: $70 \times 4.5 = 315$ grams of carbohydrate per day.

If you are very active and particularly enjoy endurance events (cycling, swimming, rowing, hillwalking, running, skiing, football, rugby, etc.), your carbohydrate requirements will be increased to 6 grams/kg body weight/day. When you increase your intake to this level, watch out for an improvement in your performance!

Table 12 gives the portions of food that will provide 50 grams of carbohydrate.

Table 12. Carbohydrate Content of Foods

Amount to provide 50 grams of carbohydrate:

Wholemeal sliced bread, large loaf	4 slices
White sliced bread, large loaf	3 slices
Oatcakes	6 round oatcakes
Malt loaf	3 slices
Hot Cross bun	2 small
Weetabix	4 biscuits
Baked potato	1 medium-sized
Wholemeal fruit scone	2 scones
Baked beans in tomato sauce	2.5 small cans

Dried figs	13
Bananas	2 large
Apple	5 large
Lentil soup	1 large bowlful
Boiled rice	2 small portions
Fresh pears	2 large
Mashed potato	4 scoops
Fresh oranges	4 medium-sized
Raisins or sultanas	5 small handfuls
Branflakes	2 medium-sized bowlfuls with skim or semi-skimmed milk
Cornflakes	2 medium-sized bowlfuls with skim or semi-skimmed milk
Pasta	70 grams (uncooked weight)

Will Exercise Affect My Appetite?

The good news for weight control is that exercise itself not only boosts metabolism during activity, but means you are essentially running on higher revs for a few hours afterwards. However, exercise also stimulates appetite, although it takes up to two hours for the effect to 'kick in'. Immediately after vigorous exercise there is an increased level of free fatty acids circulating in the blood. These were originally released from your fat stores to provide some of the energy for muscles during prolonged exercise. Until the excess is removed from the bloodstream, and re-packaged back into adipose tissue, they act as an appetite suppressor – which is why most people don't feel like eating immediately after exercise. The danger is that when your appetite does return, it is easy to overeat and put back more Calories than you have just burnt off.

One reason why exercise fails to have a significant impact on beating the bulge is because fatty foods rather than carbohydrate, are eaten after exercise. This was demonstrated in a recent study. A group of nine healthy males completed a 60-minute running session on two consecutive days (which used up approximately 500 Calories each time) and were then given free access to either low, medium or high fat foods. The results showed that when they were exposed to high-fat foods, by the end of the two days they had overeaten by 750 Calories. In contrast, the medium and low fat days resulted in undereating (–500 and –1000 Calories respectively) over the two days. This meant that it was easier to stay in energy balance, and even lose weight by choosing low fat/high carbohydrate foods after exercise.

If you choose fatty foods, the excess Calories are efficiently stored as fat on your thighs, hips or belly. Carbohydrate eaten after exercise, on the other hand, is firstly used to replenish those valuable glycogen stores – ready for the next exercise session. Once these stores have been filled, any surplus is converted to fat (unfortunately the body cannot convert fat to carbohydrate). This, as explained in Chapter 5, is an inefficient process meaning that if you do overeat, you have to take in more carbohydrate Calories before you put on weight compared with when the Calories come directly from fatty foods. Nevertheless, women still find it particularly difficult to lose weight, even when they exercise regularly. This is because the balance of hormones in a female is such that her metabolism is geared towards the storage of fat. A man doesn't have to lay down a good fat store in case of pregnancy and to provide enough energy for a subsequent period of lactation!

Fluids – The Energizing Solution

Running out of fluid is as much a cause of fatigue during exercise as running out of carbohydrate fuel. A loss of only 1 per cent of your body weight, that's around a litre of sweat, will have a dramatic effect on your performance. With less fluid in your circulation, your heart has to work harder, and everything seems more of an effort. Dehydration can reduce strength, power and endurance capacity. If you continue to lose fluid, your temperature control system starts to break down and fatigue and exhaustion sets in. All this has a simple solution – drink more! Do not rely on feeling thirsty as a guide to how much you should drink. As explained in Chapter 1, thirst is a poor indicator of our fluid needs. Get into the routine of drinking before you exercise. If you don't feel like or need a carbohydrate snack at this time, at the very least drink a large glass of water. A glass of diluted fruit juice will also give you a carbohydrate boost that is quickly absorbed.

What to Drink

The best drink to take before, during and after exercise is one that you enjoy – that way you are likely to drink more. The many sports drinks available generally fall into two types:

1. Those designed to replace fluid lost in sweat. These are the drinks which are described as hypotonic or isotonic. The former is a very dilute drink with a very low concentration of carbohydrate (around 3 per cent), some flavourings and perhaps a few vitamins and minerals. It is absorbed very quickly and is suitable to drink at any time. The word 'isotonic' simply means the same as, and in this

case the concentration of sugars and minerals is the same as our body fluids. This means that they are also absorbed very quickly, providing a small amount (5–7 per cent) of carbohydrate. They also can be drunk at any time, and compared with water they replace fluid more quickly. Isotonic drinks come pre-packaged, which is convenient but expensive. It is cheaper to make your own isotonic sports drink by mixing a litre of your favourite unsweetened fruit juice with the same amount of water and a very small pinch of salt (barely detectable when you taste the drink).

2. Energy drinks to provide a source of carbohydrate. These are hypertonic drinks as they contain much higher concentrations (around 20 per cent) of carbohydrate. This is usually in the form of glucose polymers or maltodextrins – chains of glucose molecules joined together. They allow more glucose to be packed into the same solution without it tasting unbearably sweet. Hypertonic drinks are not suitable during exercise, especially if fluid replacement is your priority. They are too concentrated, and slow down the absorption of fluid into your bloodstream. They are best used as a convenient recovery drink after strenuous exercise.

The bottom line is that people who exercise have more energy; those who don't exercise feel as though they don't want to and prefer to restrict their activity to flicking over the TV channels. Having more energy means that you not only have more energy for yourself, but for others too. If you are working long hours, striving towards your goals with great success, but your friends, family, partner or children complain that they never see you, there is something wrong with your quality of life. You are out of balance. A wobbly wheel of life certainly doesn't speed along smoothly, it lurches along until finally the spokes break and the whole machine stops. Regular exercise generates energy and helps you to sleep better. A good sleep means being able to recover and re-charge, and having more energy results in being able to spend time with others – as well as for yourself.

7

Antioxidants – Vital Defenders of Our Cells

It may seem crazy but oxygen is not only vital to life and needed to keep the embers of metabolism burning, it is also used by the body to produce incredibly toxic chemicals known as free radicals. These free radicals are constantly being generated as a normal part of metabolism, and in the last few seconds many thousands of free radicals have been produced in your body. Although they are damaging molecules they do have their uses and are harnessed by the body to destroy bacteria and virus-infected cells. They do a wonderful job, ridding the area of infection, but if they were not contained they would cause the same destruction to normal healthy cells. This is because, chemically, a free radical is a molecule which has lost one of its electrons (they are usually paired). This makes for a very unstable molecule which will try to grab an electron from another molecule in its frantic search to regain the stable paired electron state. However, if it does succeed in grabbing an electron, it leaves behind another molecule which is unstable and so the chain reaction of free radical generation continues like ripples across a pond – except that the effect is more like a bull raging through a china shop!

Since the potential damage from uncurtailed free radicals is unthinkable, the body has an in-built system designed to neutralize any wanton, unstable molecules. This system is based on molecules collectively known as antioxidants and a series of enzymes. They act to quench the chain reaction of free radical production by donating an electron – but without becoming an unstable molecule themselves. As long as the body has a sufficiently high antioxidant status, it can keep the production and damaging effects of free radicals in check. So who are these antioxidant heros? The answer is vitamins A, C and E (known as the ACE vitamins), along with beta carotene (which is converted to vitamin A in the body). These simple vitamins are the body's vital defence against the ravages of free radicals.

One of the greatest revelations in nutritional science over the last decade has been the identification of just how important the balance between free radicals and antioxidants within the body really is. There are a number of factors associated with our modern way of living that lead to the generation of higher levels of free radicals in the body. Smokers suck these particles directly into their body every time they draw on a cigarette. The gas phase of cigarette smoke contains nitric oxide and nitric dioxide, both of which can be termed free radicals as they carry an unpaired electron and are capable of initiating free radical chain reactions. It has been estimated that free radicals from one cigarette 'mop up' 0.8 mg of vitamin C. This means that a 40-a-day smoker would use 32 mg of the vitamin just in counteracting the results of his habit. Surveys of smokers' diets have shown that the average daily intake of vitamin C is an inadequate 30 mg.

Smoking has for a long time been associated with the development of emphysema, lung cancer, atherosclerosis and strokes, but the exact mechanism has remained unclear. There is now growing evidence that it is the millions of free radicals inhaled with cigarette smoke that cause the initial damage to delicate membranes. It is well known that the diet of an average smoker is not overflowing with fruit, vegetables, nuts and unprocessed cereals – the very foods which provide a good supply of the antioxidant vitamins. So, not only is the body overwhelmed with a massive onslaught of free radicals, but the antioxidant status is greatly reduced. When the body is out of balance in this way, the inevitable result is dis-ease.

In their frantic search for electrons, free radicals tear through the cell structure like gangs of muggers, leaving healthy cells distorted and destroyed. If the free radicals attack the genetic material in a cell, the codes controlling metabolism and replication are corrupted – turning a normal vibrant cell into a malignant cancerous one. No one knows the exact cause(s) of cancer, but this initial damage to the fundamental genetic code of a cell could well be an important trigger. Research papers from across the world have been flooding into the scientific journals, documenting evidence that free radical damage is an important underlying cause in many other conditions such as rheumatoid arthritis, neuro-degenerative diseases leading to poor concentration and memory loss, and coronary artery disease.

Because the free radicals wreck the basic cell structure, it is not surprising that there is such widespread damage. For example, when they attack the fatty acids in the cell membrane, the delicate structure is ripped apart turning the fat rancid and leaving the cell to die. Free radicals even attack those low density lipoproteins (the harmful LDLs), already not exactly flavour of the month. Recent research has shown that once the free radicals have turned the fat in an LDL particle rancid, it is more likely to be deposited in the artery wall and lead to atherosclerosis. The LDL particle does actually contain a small supply of vitamin E and beta carotene but these antioxidants are overwhelmed by the damaging effects of cigarette smoke.

It is not only smokers who are under free radical attack. Pollution and car exhaust fumes which clog the air of any busy city also provide extra free radicals, as do pesticide chemicals in foods, radiation during air travel and from computer screens, microwave ovens, electric blankets, tanning beds, television sets, x-rays, radios, high voltage wiring in overhead pylons and fluorescent lighting. A high-fat diet and exposure to sunlight (UV radiation) also result in increased free radical generation. Also, whilst there is no doubt that regular activity has tremendous health benefits, it does involve increased metabolism, and the natural by-product of this is free radical production. Nevertheless, many of the high carbohydrate foods (wholemeal bread, dried apricots, salad and root vegetables, bananas and other fresh fruits) which provide the right type of fuel for exercise, also supply the body with extra antioxidant vitamins and minerals.

Think about the list of factors which contribute to the total free radical load that you receive. Add up the daily exposure you get from all of these and you'll see how significant free radical attack can be. You will be pleased to learn that you can eat your way out of this dilemma! You can provide your body with foods bursting with beta carotene and vitamins A, C and E and flood each cell with antioxidant compounds that will intercept and neutralize the rampaging free radicals – and even repair some of their damage.

Get Some Colour In Your Diet

Beta carotene, a similar carotenoid substance called lycopene (which is responsible for the red colour of tomatoes), the ACE vitamins and the minerals selenium, zinc and copper play an important role in the quenching of free radicals.

When you eat foods which contain these, the antioxidants infuse into each cell where they act as the main fire fighters and take the heat out of any free radical attack. Fruits and vegetables, especially carrots, broccoli, spinach, lettuce, tomatoes, oranges, kiwi fruits, blackcurrants, peaches, mangoes, papaya, water melon and Cantaloup melon are the best sources of beta carotene, lycopene, vitamins A and C and some of the minerals. As a general rule, the darker the colour of carrots, oranges or peaches and the deeper green of lettuce, broccoli or cabbage the higher the vitamin content. Since colour is a powerful factor which makes us choose to eat a food, it is time to banish those artificial ones added to processed foods and relish the natural colours in foods. Let colour be your guide to eating foods which not only look good but have the awesome power to protect against free radicals. Almonds, peanuts, hazel nuts, sunflower seeds, olive oil, avocado pears, and wholemeal bread are not so highly coloured but are wonderful sources of vitamin E.

The Fresh Way to Beat Nicotine Craving

Every year thousands of people make a crucial decision that will change their lives and boost their health – they decide to give up smoking, and many of them succeed. It's reassuring that the harmful effects of smoking on health can be cleared within five years of kicking the habit. Hypnosis has an impressively high success rate (around 80 per cent in some clinics) in helping people give up, but what is less well publicized is the fact that antioxidants have a vital role to play in resisting the weed. They can energize your body and really launch you into your new life as a non-smoker. It works like this. Once you have stopped smoking, there is still the addictive nicotine in your system which fuels the craving to reach for a new packet. One remedy is to use a nicotine patch. These feed the addiction, without your having to reach for a cigarette, but are not a long term solution. Although it may not seem like it when you're giving up, nicotine clears from the body quite rapidly. Residual nicotine is reduced by around 50 per cent after three days, and after three weeks the body is 99 per cent free of the toxin. The trick is to get through the first three weeks of detoxification – but what you eat during this time can have a significant effect on whether you succeed.

Having stubbed out their last cigarette, many people turn to bars of chocolate, packets of crisps and sweets for consolation or reward. These are low nutrient density foods, lacking in those vital antioxidants – which, remember, have been very much drained by the effects of cigarette smoke. Chances are that ex-smokers may be suffering from a mild deficiency of several vitamins. It is easy to confuse the symptoms of these deficiencies – fatigue, headaches, jangling nerves, irritability, muscle weakness, susceptibility to colds and flu, pale pasty skin – with what is 'normal' for a smoker, or the effects of giving up. All of this can be prevented and the detoxification phase speeded up by bombarding your body with the antioxidant nutrients. This means reaching for a piece of fruit every time you get a craving to eat. Dried apricots, raisins, figs, prunes and dates are good to nibble on, and if you need to keep your hands occupied – peel an orange!

The World Health Organization's slogan 'Five-a-Day' reminds us to reach daily for five portions of fruits and vegetables (potatoes don't count), equivalent to 1 lb a day. This is no problem when summer fruits, such as strawberries, cantaloup melons, peaches, nectarines and mangoes, dazzle us with colour and flavour. But in winter it's not so easy. So, for those who struggle to eat their pound of fruit and vegetable flesh, isn't the solution to be found in vitamin supplementation to boost their antioxidant status? There is no doubt that supplements do have their uses, and are convenient when we are away from our normal routine of eating an array of fruit and vegetables. There are also times in our lives when there is an increased requirement for specific nutrients. Women who intend to become pregnant should aim to supplement their daily diet or eat foods (liver, dark green vegetables, melons, dried apricots), particularly rich in iron and folic acid. Mature women who are not exposed to much sunlight can benefit from cod liver oil capsules as a source of vitamin D. Also, at times of high stress multi-B-vitamin supplementation is justified.

However, these individual nutrient supplements simply cannot replicate the power of nature's natural vitamin larder – whole foods. For example, in nature there are four different chemical forms of vitamin E. Vitamin tablets only contain one of these forms. In addition, scientists have been discovering a whole world of bio-active compounds in plant foods, collectively known as phytochemicals. The exact role of these substances has yet to be detailed, but in time they may turn out to be even more important than the 'big three' ACE antioxidant nutrients. Only time will tell, but right now only real foods provide this complete spectrum of phytochemicals. As research techniques advance we must not lose sight of the whole picture. Nutrients are placed in foods for a purpose. They work together, and their action can be compromised by the absence of one of the team members. A vitamin pill or concentrate may be a high tech, no fuss, convenient way of swallowing the vital substances that we know about, but at present it is impossible to replicate perfectly and to jam the range and fine balance of nutrients found in foods into a capsule.

The Magic of Tea, Red Wine and Onions!

Once the awesome potential power of free radicals to promote disease and the potential of antioxidants to prevent them had been realized, scientists began analysing foods for those phytochemicals and other substances that may have antioxidant properties. The search has turned up a number of other compounds, including quercetin, kaempferol, myricetin, apigenin and luteolin. The list goes on, but they can all be lumped under the name of flavonoids. This is a large group of naturally occurring polyphenolic antioxidants which are found not only in fruits and vegetables but also in drinks such as tea and wine.

The antioxidant power of both black (fermented) and green (unfermented) tea is easy to demonstrate in a test tube, but a recent study showed that the same effect occurs in the body. Volunteers drank either black or green tea or water after an overnight fast before the antioxidant activity in their blood was measured. Results showed that there was a significant rise in this after tea drinking against no change when water was drunk. It was also found that adding milk to the tea reduced the antioxidant power. It seems that the milk proteins form complexes with the polyphenols, and these are not absorbed into the body. The message, then, is to drink black tea with lemon instead of milk – a refreshing drink which can be enjoyed cold in the summer. Green tea has the added advantage over black tea in that it is much lower in caffeine. A major inter-university study in Japan has found that green tea can help to reduce blood pressure in those who suffer from hypertension. Other studies have produced evidence that the polyphenol compounds found in both green and black tea have an important role in preventing some cancers – especially cancer of the skin, lung, stomach and colon. Surprisingly, cancer of the oesophagus is particularly high in some Middle Eastern countries where tea drinking is very popular. It has been suggested that the cancer probably results from the scalding temperature at which the tea is drunk! It is well known that tea is naturally rich in the mineral fluoride, which helps to prevent tooth decay.

To enhance a fine meal, your health and your enjoyment, sip a few glasses of red wine. In 1990 French scientists reported that volunteers who drank half a litre of red wine a day for two weeks significantly increased not only their levels of HDL (the 'good' cholesterol), but their antioxidant status as well. When the volunteers switched to white wine and other forms of alcohol, there was no such benefit. Red wine contains a number of those phenolic compounds, including a natural fungicide called resveratrol. This is found on grape skins which, to make red wine, are crushed to a pulp and fermented. The method used to make white wine is slightly different. Here the grapes are crushed, but the grape juice is fermented rather than the pulp. Some red wines from Bordeaux have been found to have 200 times the phenol content of most white wines. These have a powerful antioxidant effect but, unlike tea drinking, more is certainly not better!

Onions and Garlic

For many years, onions and garlic have been known to have anti-inflammatory, anti-bacterial, anti-fungal action. They are one of nature's true miracle medicines and we are just beginning to understand why. Onions are an incredibly rich source of quercetin, one of the most biologically active members of the flavonoid antioxidants. It seems to act in conjunction with the immune system and helps to inhibit the release of histamine from cells and so dampen the effects of pollen in hay fever and other allergies. Quercetin also helps to prevent the formation of blood clots and so reduce the risk of stroke. The best source of quercetin is onions – but choose the yellow or red ones, as white onions have a poor quercetin content.

Surprisingly, garlic, which is a close family member to onions, does not contain quercetin. It does, however, have at least 10 other antioxidant chemicals, and their activity in the body is probably the key to garlic's health-giving properties. Garlic tops the American National Cancer Institute's list of cancer-preventing foods. It also helps to relieve bloating and to control diarrhoea. Garlic contains an anti-coagulant substance called ajoene which helps to thin the blood and prevent it from clotting. Other substances have been identified which have been found to inhibit the production of cholesterol in the liver which then helps to control blood cholesterol levels. Raw garlic is best for its anti-bacterial activity, but cooking does not diminish garlic's other effects. However, the powers of garlic are lost when it is powdered or used as garlic salt.

Antioxidants – How Much Do I Need?

How many antioxidants you need to best support your health and boost the vitality of every cell in your body will depend on a number of factors in your life. Remember the function of antioxidants is to neutralize the free radicals which are either produced within your body or taken in from the environment. You need to add up your free radical stresses. The more of the following that apply to you, the higher your intake of antioxidants (from all food and drink sources) should be.

- Living in a city – air pollution.
- Regular air travel.
- Tobacco smoke – including passive smoking.
- Regular exposure to sunlight.
- Vigorous, frequent exercise.
- Over the age of 50.
- Working daily with computers, microwave ovens, near electricity pylons.
- Daily exposure to fluorescent lighting.
- Stress which you feel that you cannot control either at home or at work.

At the very least, aim to eat five servings of highly coloured vegetables or fruit every day. If you have several of the free radical stresses, top up each day your 'Five-A-Day' with:
- Six cups of weak black or green China tea, without milk.
- Half an onion – cooked or in salads.
- 3 cloves of garlic.
- 2 glasses of red wine (depending on your alcohol tolerance).
- 1 Avocado.

Antioxidant Food File

Foods Rich in All Three Antioxidant, ACE, Vitamins

Broccoli, tomatoes, red and green peppers, spinach, watercress, brussels sprouts, sweet potatoes, mango, guavas, kale, lettuce.

Foods Rich in Vitamin C

Strawberries, blackcurrants, Kiwi fruit, oranges, lemons, limes, grapefruit, parsley.

Foods Rich in Vitamin A (as Beta-carotene)

Carrots, Cantaloupe melons, apricots, pumpkin, turnip, yellow peppers.

Foods Rich in Vitamin E

Avocado pear, cold-pressed extra virgin olive oil, green and black olives, sunflower seeds, tahini (sesame seed paste rather like peanut butter), walnuts.

8

Making Changes

The key to making changes of any sort is first to change what is between your ears. Control of your mind must come first because your mind controls your body. What you eat is a symbol of what you believe. There is no magic cure for poor eating habits, but you can change the way you eat by changing the way you think. If you believe that there is a list of 'good' and 'bad' foods (and that the latter comes with the ambivalent mix of pleasure and guilt), or that exercise is a chore and you have to suffer to get fit or lose a bit of weight – then so it all will be.

It is important to transform your thinking from the negative and self-defeating images of yourself to positive, optimistic ones. In the same way that success in business stems from the power of positive thinking, if you change your attitude towards food and believe that moderation not martyrdom is the key, you release yourself from the fear of food and the 'naughty but nice' mentality. You then begin to see food for what it is – your ultimate energy advantage which fuels your body and feeds your mind and which, at the same time, can be enjoyed, savoured and relished.

Think Yourself Thin, Fit, Happy and Energized

One powerful yet simple strategy to help you achieve this is creative visualization. This is a widely-used discipline both in business and in world class sport. By seeing yourself as you would like to be, you establish in your mind a clear image of your goal. For instance, before a tournament, many of the top golfers will 'see' themselves lining up a difficult put and sinking the ball successfully. The same technique can help you change your self-image and your attitude to food – or indeed anything you wish to achieve.

The first thing you need to do is to make yourself comfortable, and concentrate on your breathing. This will help you to relax so that you can empty your mind of all intruding thoughts. It is vital to clear your mind. This is quite a challenge at first, as random thoughts persist, but it becomes easier as you progress. Now, form an image of yourself as you would like to be – lean, slim, fit, in control, full of confidence with plenty of energy. Picture yourself in your own house getting dressed to go out. Notice how well your clothes fit – none of the tight waistband of the 'old you'. Check yourself in the mirror and compliment yourself on your appearance. Now open the front door and walk outside. Notice how well you feel as the new you – with a lightness, vitality and spring in your step. Form an image of the people you meet along the way and hear them comment on the fact that you have lost weight and that you look fantastic. Relish the boost to your self-esteem that it gives you, and feel yourself growing taller.

Build these visualization sessions (20 minutes a day) into your life. Pretty soon you will begin to feel like the new you. What's more you may find that your eating habits have changed. Maybe you find that whereas before, after a nice meal in a restaurant, you always made room for dessert. Now for no obvious reason, and certainly not through an enormous display of will-power, you decline what is on offer. In essence, you have begun to eat like the slimmer, fitter person that you want to be – but without the feelings of denial that you might previously have associated with the so-called 'forbidden foods'. As you practise, the images become bigger and more powerful and have an even greater effect on your everyday behaviour.

The Power of the Right Brain

The success of creative visualization lies in the mind's unique ability to think in two separate ways. The brain has two hemispheres, left and right, which are designed to process information in very different ways. The left brain deals with the logical thinking which allows us to understand mathematics, technology and engineering or learn a language, whilst the right brain is for creativity, emotional and intuitive thinking. One of the effects of caffeine is to stimulate the left brain, which is why heavy coffee drinkers can stay awake all night dealing with mundane, routine, logical tasks, but their potential for original thought and problem solving is stunted.

The right brain has great potential for those who know how to use it. Experts agree that there are three basic methods for stimulating right brain activity: creative visualization, drawing pictures and sleeping well. If this seems illogical or a bit simplistic, it is because you are using your left brain now! Creative visualization, forming positive images in your mind allows your right brain to work *for*, rather than *against* you. As Aristotle so accurately said, 'The soul never thinks without a picture.' We now know that imagery is the basis of our thought processes. The brain does not recognize words, so communicate with your right brain by visual images. This process can be enhanced by drawing pictures. This is how the mind-mapping techniques, pioneered by Tony Buzan, help business teams by combining their logic and organizational skills with problem solving and creative thinking.

An effective method for coming up with a solution to a problem is to 'sleep on it'. However, rather than spending a restless night agonizing, the trick is to feed your left brain with information, then let go. During the periods of REM sleep, your right brain takes over and sometime later, as if in a flash of inspiration, the solution is at hand. As explained in Chapter 2, caffeine interferes with REM sleep and so reduces the potential of your right brain to provide the solutions to the challenges of everyday life.

Take Control of Your Own Health Now

What motivates us to change? Usually it is a crisis, an illness – heart attack, diabetes, stroke, cancer, ulcer. Why not take stock, and put health and energy at the top of your agenda NOW. Now is the time when, if you choose to take control, you have plenty of options to regain your lost energy and to improve your health. Once you have become seriously ill, you have lost control over your health. The options then tend to pass to your doctor, who may be able to patch up the effects of years of neglect. Delegation is fine, but don't delegate your health. You must make the change and discard the patch-up approach that most people adopt to cope with life.

Table 13. Destructive and Constructive Strategies

Patch-up destructive strategy	What you want	What you get
Reaching for processed, concentrated sugary snacks	Energy	Temporary high then a crashing low
Excess alcohol	Relaxation/sedation	Depression
Drinking coffee/Colas	Stimulation	Fatigue
Eating fast foods	Quick re-fuelling	Indigestion, fatigue, overweight
Comfort eating	Sedation, escape	Masking of symptoms, illness, fatigue, guilt
Fake fats and artificial sweeteners	Calorie-controlled diet	Confused appetite control, compensatory eating, overweight, relying on food which takes the guilt but also the pleasure out of eating

Constructive Strategies	What you want	What you get
Cutting down/ giving up caffeine	Mental energy	Mental energy, creative thinking, calmness, a good night's sleep
Fruit snacks	Mental and physical boost	Sustained blood sugar level, energizing antioxidants
Taking a breather	Relaxation	Re-charged and re-vitalized
Sleeping well	To be refreshed	Refreshed, calm and in control

Regular exercise	Fitness	Mental and physical fitness; renewed vigour; stamina; improved self-esteem, joint flexibility, strength and co-ordination; less anxiety; levels of antibodies which help to combat infection increase by 20 per cent; skin improves – becomes stronger, thicker and more elastic
Taking time to chew foods and choosing foods that need chewing	Improved digestion	Improved digestion and inner health. Relief from wind, bloating, constipation
Eating quality foods	Increased enjoyment	Enjoyment and quality nutrition

Small Changes – Big Results

Most human beings don't like change – it can be unsettling and threaten security, and making a major change to your lifestyle is no exception. The secret of success is to make the change bit by bit. Just as a climb to the summit of Everest begins with a single step, overhauling your eating patterns begins with a single meal. You don't have to revamp your whole diet overnight. Tossing out a set of habits that have taken a lifetime to form is too much of a wrench to the system, which is why that approach doesn't work. Just one small permanent change is better than all the crash diet attempts put together.

So, if you have doubts about the value of the extra time needed to shop, prepare or choose food against the existing demands on life, if good nutrition seems like too much of an effort, it is time to narrow your scope. The case of the overworked accountant proves this point. He didn't have time to think about food, so always ate the same – an extra-large hamburger and a large portion of french fries – five days a week for lunch. He was persuaded by a nutritionist to eat a small hamburger and a small portion of fries twice a week and tuna fish sandwiches on the other days. He lost 1 lb a week because the change saved him a total of 3,500 calories and 125 grams of fat. After 10 weeks he had lost 10 lb and his total blood cholesterol level and blood pressure were normalized – all from making one single change!

The first step, then, is to decide on and concentrate upon one particular change. Here are some suggestions:

- Cut down on or eliminate caffeine-containing drinks and foods. If you rely on a vending machine at the office for drinks, make sure the caterers stock it with a decaffeinated option.
- Take your own lunchtime snack and take a break from work to eat it. Enjoy thick vegetable soups with chunks of wholemeal bread in the winter; filled rolls and fruits (melon, strawberries, peaches, nectarines, plums) in the summer. Spread your sandwiches or bread with half as much butter.
- Enjoy business lunches, but eat like the French. Start the meal with a serving of vegetables with crusty bread. You will have more energy and probably impress your client or colleague with your eating habits!
- In the office canteen, replace at least one meat meal per week with one based on oily fish (mackerel, salmon, sardines, trout, etc.).

- If you eat at a local sandwich shop, choose low-fat fillings such as tuna salad, spicy chicken, prawn or egg salad, and avoid those which include mayonnaise. Ask for butter on one side of the bread only and plenty of lettuce, chopped radish, onion, cucumber, tomato, etc.
- Take a mid-morning or afternoon break and enjoy a snack, but replace your usual chocolate bar every now and then with a piece (or several pieces) of fruit. Eventually, eating fruit rather than sugar will become a habit.
- Eat an avocado instead of a cheese-based dish once a week.
- Adjust the size of the portions of foods you eat so that you shift the balance and choose fewer of the fatty foods and more of the starchy carbohydrate ones. For example, if you always have a cheese sandwich for lunch, cut the bread slices much thicker and the cheese much thinner. Enjoy mountains of pasta or rice with less of the cheese, meat or curry sauce. Choose a deep pan pizza with less cheese and meat topping rather than a thin base smothered with these.
- Opt for the real thing, don't settle for fake fats or artificial sweeteners. If you drink a lot of diet drinks, wean these out and replace them with more fruit juices (diluting them with soda water makes a refreshing long drink), herb teas and mineral water.
- Put bread back on your menu – and work up to six slices a day. Choose wholemeal or good quality white bread, that you would enjoy eating six slices of, from a local or traditional baker. Better still, try making it yourself (kneading the dough is so therapeutic!). The mass-produced, soft, white sliced loaf available in the UK has been stripped of any nutritional value and is an insult to the senses.
- Several of the major airlines offer special meals which are low in salt, sugar and dairy ingredients. These must be

booked in advance. British Airways have a 'Raid the Larder' alternative on some flights where you are invited to select a snack from a display of foods instead of having a full meal. Choose plenty of fruit and ask for extra water so that you arrive at your destination well hydrated and ready to do business.

Once your new food or routine has become as automatic as brushing your teeth, add in one more and just keep going. It takes 21 days to establish a new habit, so be patient. Remember the Gucci principle that long after the cost is forgotten, the quality remains. It is the direction of change that is important, not the speed. Keep visualizing, keep the image of the person you want to be clear in your mind.

If you try to make one of the mini changes listed earlier and it doesn't work for you, then try something else. Most of us have the wrong approach to success; when we don't achieve something we try harder – over and over again. What distinguishes highly successful people is that when they don't succeed, they try something else.

Emotional Eating and Comfort Foods

Sometimes a poor diet is a symptom of a larger problem. Many people have lost touch with real hunger and suffer from 'emotional hunger'. They use food to satisfy their feelings rather than their 'body hunger' and physiological need for energy and nutrients. Do you eat when you are bored, lonely, tired, upset, angry? With so much stress in the workplace, it is easy to use food to numb your emotions and escape from the pressures in the office – at least for a short while.

Food then serves as a comforter – which is not surprising since when we were young and we cried, we were often pacified with something to eat. As adults, food brings the same consolation – but the effect is only temporary. If you can't seem to fill yourself with food, then food may not be what you really want. A lot of people confuse tiredness for hunger and push snacks into their mouths when a break or a good night's sleep is the real solution. Don't use food as a tranquillizer. Have you become convinced that the only way to survive and get through the day is with the help of a packet of digestive biscuits?

Gorging food may serve to numb our emotions but this can lead to guilt – which only adds to the negative view we have of ourselves. This route leads to obesity and eating disorders. To control emotional eating, keep a food diary and use it to identify the danger zones. Figure out the reasons why you eat what you eat and the times that you eat. Some people confuse hunger with every other feeling or excuse under the sun. Others use food to fill in the gaps between everything they do: the gap between arriving home from work and being at home; the gap between changing from one activity to another; the gap between television programmes. If you want to change your emotional eating patterns, you need to change your life and get to the underlying cause of your emotions. Changing your eating habits at a time when emotions rule what and how much food you put in your mouth is hopeless. Remember the saying: 'It is difficult to remember to drain the swamp when you are up to your neck in crocodiles!'

Using sheer willpower to deprive yourself of the foods that your emotional state craves will not work. Simply screwing your eyes closed and mentally shouting 'no, no, no!' every time you find yourself moving towards the kitchen or nearest supermarket is not the solution. The conflict is between your left brain providing you with rational, logical reasons why you don't need to eat and your right brain full of your emotional needs. A real contest is on. Your rational mind says cottage cheese sandwich when, to your much more powerful emotional mind, only a bowl of ice cream and cheesecake will do. Guess who wins?

In this situation, you cannot change by rational thought alone. If you could, you would have done it by now. You need to short-circuit the programme which drives you to eat when you are not hungry and replace it with a new programme that will provide you with alternatives. When you are tired, take a break. When you are bored, do something else that is pleasurable apart from eating. Learning to address and answer your real needs is much more of a challenge than simply reaching for food as an anaesthetic. Unless you confront the underlying problem, it will not go away. A boring job will still be boring no matter how many cream cakes you eat.

Plan for Tomorrow but Live for Today

It is time to develop a new enthusiasm for life and take responsibility for your own well-being. Ask yourself if you are happy? Do you look forward to work, enjoy a good social life, feel relaxed, energized and carefree? If the answer is 'not really' then it is time to make changes.

Do you really want to look back on your life wishing that you had achieved more of your business goals, spent more time with your family and friends or had the energy to cram just a little more fun into each day. Instead we get stuck in a rut, busying ourselves with boring, mundane tasks that we are convinced are important. In short, most of us spend too much time surviving and too little time actually living and enjoying life. Then it's over and that's a shame.

Psychologist Srully Blotnick strongly supports the idea that enthusiasm and passion are essential to personal achievement. In 1960, Blotnick began following the lives of 1,500 people; 20 years later 1,067 were still in the study and 83 had become millionaires. In his book *Getting Rich Your Own Way* he describes this research, and without exception the millionaires cited persistence as their greatest asset – but a closer look suggests that their real secret was their passion.

If you follow the principles and at least make some of the changes described in this book, you will gain the energy advantage. Eating well gives you the stamina and confidence to take risks, face your fears and to benefit from the fine art of daring. It gives you the capacity to live in the NOW – as if each day were your last.

Further Reading

Black, Jack. *Mindstore: The Ultimate Mental Fitness Programme* , Thorsons, 1994.

Blythman, Joanna. *The Food We Eat*, Michael Joseph, 1996.

Buzan, Tony. *Using Your Head: Mind Mapping* BBC Books, 1974.

Canfield, Jack and Hansen, Mark Victor. *Dare to Win*, Berkley Books, New York, 1996.

Colclough, Beechy. *It's Not What You Eat, It's Why You Eat, It* Vermillion, 1995.

Douillard, John. *Body, Mind and Sport: The Mind-Body Guide to Lifelong Fitness and Your Personal Best*, Bantam Books, 1994.

Edwards, Betty. *Drawing On the Right Side of the Brain*, Harper-Collins, 1993.

Jackson, Adam. *The Secrets of Abundant Happiness*, Thorsons, 1996.

Katz, Donald. *Just Do It: The Nike Spirit in a Corporate*, World Adams Publishing, 1996.

Lavie, Peretz. *The Enchanting World of Sleep*, Yale, 1996.

Matthews, Andrew, *Being Happy: A Handbook to Greater Confidence and Security*, Media Masters, 1988.

McGannon, Dr Michael. *The Urban Warrior's Book of Solutions: Staying Healthy, Fit and Sane in the Business Jungle*, Pitman, 1996.

Rossi, Ernest and Nimmons, David. *The 20 Minute Break: Using the Science of Ultradian Rhythms*, Jeremy P. Tarcher, 1991.

Index